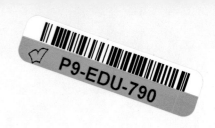

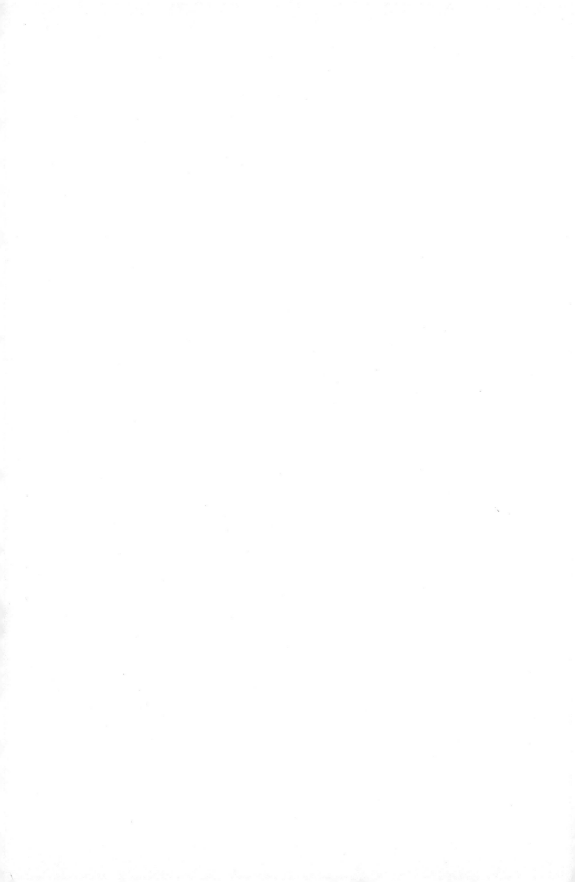

Strength Fitness

Physiological Principles and Training Techniques

EXPANDED SECOND EDITION

WAYNE L. WESTCOTT, PH.D.

ALLYN AND BACON, INC.
Boston London Sydney Toronto

For my wife, Claudia, and my parents, Warren and Eva Westcott

Credits

Part of the preface reprinted by permission from Wayne L. Westcott, "Instructor Training Key To YMCA Fitness Leadership," *Journal of Physical Education and Program*, September, 1985. Parts of Chapter Six reprinted by permission from Wayne L. Westcott, "The Case For Slow Strength Training Technique," *Scholastic Coach*, August 1984.

Library of Congress Cataloging-in-Publication Data

Westcott, Wayne L., 1949–
  Strength fitness.

  Bibliography: p.
  Includes index.
  1. Muscle strength. 2. Exercise—Physiological
aspects. 3. Physical fitness. 4. Physical education
and training. I. Title.
QP321.W44   1987   613.7′1   87-1449
ISBN 0-205-10493-2

Printed in the United States of America

10 9 8 7 6 5 4 3 2 1 92 91 90 89 88 87

Contents

Preface   vii

Chapter One
Benefits of Strength Training   1

Improved Physical Appearance   1
Improved Physical Capacity   2
Improved Athletic Performance   3
Improved Metabolic Function   4
Reduced Risk of Injury   5
Reaching One's Strength Potential   6

Chapter Two
Physiology of Strength Development · 11

Muscle Structure   11
Muscle Physiology   13
Muscle Contraction   13
Muscle Force   15
Fiber Types   18
Muscle Relaxation   19
Muscle Function   20

Chapter Three
Factors That Affect Strength Performance   27

Biomechanical Factors   27
Size Factors   31
Sex Factors   34
Age Factors   36
Training Experience   37
Training Technique   39
Training Specificity   40
Alarm   41
Muscle Stretch   41

iii

Chapter Four

Principles of Strength Training   43

Principle of Stress Adaptation   44
Principle of Rebuilding Time   46
Principle of Near-Maximum Resistance   50
Principle of Controlled Movement Speed   51
Principle of Full-Range Movements   52
Principle of Muscle Balance   54
Principle of Training Specificity   56
Summary of Training Principles   58

Chapter Five

Research on Strength Training   61

Effects of Different Training Frequencies on
    Strength Development   62
Effects of Different Training Sets on Strength
    Development   65
Effects of Different Training Repetitions on
    Strength Development   73
Effects of Different Training Speeds on Strength
    Development   76
Effects of Different Training Times on Strength
    Development   79
Effects of Strength Training on Blood Pressure   81
Effects of Strength Training on Heart Rate   88
Effects of Strength Training on Cardiovascular
    Performance   90
Effects of Strength Training on Muscle Performance   93
Effects of Strength Training on Body Composition   96
Summary of Research on Strength Training   98

Chapter Six

Designing the Strength Training Program   101

Exercise Selection   101
Exercise Frequency   105
Exercise Duration   107
Exercise Intensity   109

Exercise Speed   111
Exercise Range   116
Exercise Progression   118
Exercise Continuity   120
Summary of Program Design   121

Chapter Seven

Strength Training Considerations   *123*

Training Safety   123
Training Partners   129
Training Equipment   131
Activity Integration   143

Chapter Eight

Strength Training Exercises   *147*

Quadriceps   147
Hamstrings   151
Hip Adductors   152
Hip Abductors   152
Low Back   154
Abdominals   155
Chest   158
Upper Back   160
Shoulders   167
Triceps   170
Biceps   173
Neck Flexors   176
Neck Extensors   177
Calves   178
Forearms   180
Trapezius   180

Chapter Nine

Questions About Strength Training   *183*

What Results Should One Expect?   183
How Should One Assess Progress?   186
How Should One Deal with Strength Plateaus?   188

Should One Follow a Special Diet?   190

How Does Strength Training Affect Body Composition?   195

How Does Strength Training Affect Flexibility?   197

How Does Strength Training Affect Speed, Power, and
    Sports Performance?   198

How Do Women Respond to Strength Training?   202

How Do Persons over Thirty Respond to Strength
    Training?   203

What About Warm-Ups and Cool-Downs?   205

What Is the Relationship between Muscle Strength
    and Muscle Size?   208

What Is the Relationship between Muscle Strength
    and Muscle Endurance?   209

What Is the Relationship between Muscle Strength
    and Cardiovascular Endurance?   211

Appendix A

Strength Training Equipment   215

Appendix B

Principles of Force Production   217

Appendix C

*Training Effects of Endurance Exercise
    upon the Cardiovascular System   219*

Appendix D

Strength Training Checklist   223

Appendix E

Strength Training Logbook   225

Glossary   227
Bibliography   235
Index   241

Preface

Not many years ago, two books had a profound impact on the lifestyles of millions of Americans. *Aerobics* by Kenneth Cooper, and *The Official YMCA Physical Fitness Handbook,* by Clayton Myers, motivated men and women from all walks of life to pursue regular physical activity. Both books emphasized large muscle activities of an aerobic nature. The intent was to improve the cardiovascular condition of our adult population and to reduce the incidence of coronary heart disease.

The YMCA program centered on group activity, including group fitness testing, group fitness orientation, and group fitness classes. It was highly successful because cardiovascular exercise was new and people wanted professionally supervised activity sessions.

Cooper's protocol was designed more for the individual exerciser. Participants scored points for performing a variety of aerobic activities such as jogging, cycling, swimming, and walking. As more and more fitness information was published, the popularity of at-home exercise increased. People cycled to work, walked during their lunch hours, and jogged before breakfast when the environment was peaceful and cool.

The aerobic phenomenon fostered a new lifestyle that quickly gained acceptance by physicians, physical educators, and the general public. However, the long-term results of the aerobic movement were both predictable and unpredictable, good and bad. For the better, the aerobic exercisers experienced increased cardiovascular fitness and decreased risk of heart disease. For the worse, more than 50 percent of the joggers and aerobic dancers developed musculoskeletal injuries and were forced to discontinue their training programs. This was because the repetitive, mid-range movements involved in these endurance activities caused the muscles to develop in an unbalanced manner.

Ironically, the very activities that improved cardiovascular function in thousands of adults created an epidemic of overuse injuries and ushered in the era of sports medicine. Apparently, in our well-intentioned quest for cardiovascular fitness we forgot about the musculoskeletal system. The solution is not to give up aerobic activities, but to perform appropriate muscle strengthening exercises for all of the major muscle groups to insure balanced musculoskeletal development.

There is considerable misunderstanding about strength training and musculoskeletal development. Young men are afraid they won't have enough muscle, and young women are afraid they will have too much.

Strength training can increase muscle strength, muscle density, and muscle tone, but may have little influence on muscle size. Muscle size is largely determined by inherited factors. Very few women have the genetic potential to develop large muscles, and most men must learn to be content with a moderate musculature.

Actually, almost every human activity requires coordinated muscle movement. Muscles are just as important for speaking, writing, and playing a guitar as for running, swimming, and lifting weights. Although thinking uses a small amount of energy, most of our energy supplies are consumed by large muscle activity. Muscle maintenance also requires a considerable amount of energy. Other things being equal, a person in good muscular condition will have a higher rate of calorie utilization than a person in poor muscular condition.

So what is the purpose of strength training? Simply, it is to improve muscle function, to look better, to feel better, to move better, to utilize calories better, to work better, to play better, to reduce the risk of injury, and to delay the degenerative processes that are a natural part of aging.

Strength training can be performed with barbells at home or with Nautilus equipment at a YMCA. The most important thing in beginning a strength training program is competent instruction. The following chapters provide relevant information regarding strength training principles and practices that should be part of the instructional process.

Acknowledgments

The author acknowledges the invaluable assistance of Dr. Ellington Darden, Mr. James Flanagan, Dr. Ted Lambrinides, Mr. Joseph Martino, Mr. George Ramsden, Mr. Ralph Yohe, Mr. Donald Brownell, and Mr. Paul Harvey. Special appreciation is extended to Mrs. Leslie Willis who provided all the photographs and illustrations, and to Mrs. Claudia Westcott who typed the manuscript for this text.

Chapter One

Benefits of Strength Training

IMPROVED PHYSICAL APPEARANCE

There are a number of benefits that result from proper strength training, but the most obvious is improved physical appearance. In fact, the principal reason that most people begin a strength training program is to look better. Looking fit is basically a matter of muscle tone, and muscle tone is closely related to muscle strength.

Consider the average American woman with a bodyweight of approximately 135 pounds. In terms of body composition, bones account for about 15 pounds, organs and skin account for about 35 pounds, fat accounts for about 35 pounds, and muscle contributes about 50 pounds. Although too much fat can certainly detract from one's appearance, it is the muscle tissue that really determines one's body contours. Those 50 pounds of muscle provide the raw material for developing a pleasing and symmetrical shape.

There is some confusion regarding the relationship of muscle strength, muscle tone, and muscle size. As muscle strength improves, muscle tone improves due to greater density of the muscle fibers. Everyone can increase muscle strength and muscle tone to some degree. However, very few men and even fewer women have the genetic potential to develop large muscles. During the past decade, many adults have come to understand these concepts through regular participation in strength training programs. Few have developed large muscles, but most have experienced improved muscle strength, improved muscle tone, and improved physical appearance. That is why strength training is currently one of the most popular adult physical activities.

Strength training is somewhat unique in that the results are readily apparent to the exerciser and others. Improvements in muscle strength and physical appearance are usually noticeable after four weeks of training, and these visible reinforcers provide excellent motivation to continue one's exercise program.

IMPROVED PHYSICAL CAPACITY

Perhaps the most dramatic result of proper strength training is the large increase in one's capacity to perform work. Previously untrained men normally experience about 40 percent improvement in muscle performance after one month of strength training. Although some of the initial increase is due to more coordinated execution of the exercise movement, participants are invariably impressed with the results. These positive physical changes give excellent incentive to pursue further training, even when the strength gains come more slowly.

In accordance with the principle of stress adaptation (see Chapter 4), progressive strength training provides the stimulus for numerous physiological adaptations. Within the muscle, there is an increase in fiber density and improvements in protein synthesis, energy production, and blood distribution, all of which contribute to better physical performance.

Because muscle strength and muscle endurance are so closely related, more muscle strength results in more muscle endurance at any given workload. That is, strength training enables one to work harder and longer at a particular exercise level, and to perform previously difficult tasks with much less effort.

It is important to understand that every physical activity requires a certain percentage of one's maximum muscle strength. For persons with little muscle strength, typical household chores such as snow shoveling, grocery carrying, and gardening can be physically demanding activities. As they become stronger, these same tasks will require a lower percentage of their available muscle strength and thus be much easier to perform.

Muscle strength is basic to human function. If we compare the human body to an automobile, the muscles are analogous to the engine, and the heart serves as the fuel pump. The fuel pump is very important, but the car won't move if the engine is in bad shape. In recent years, we have placed much emphasis on conditioning the cardiovascular system. It is time we realized that to be physically fit one must have strong muscles as well as a strong heart.

IMPROVED ATHLETIC PERFORMANCE

Successful sports performance is largely dependent upon the athlete's ability to produce power. Almost every athletic event has a power component. Power is most evident in activities such as putting a shot, punting a football, hitting a baseball, dunking a basketball, and sprinting 100 yards. But power is also involved in running a five-mile race. Assuming similar bodyweights, all of the racers perform the same amount of work. The winner, however, performs the work in the least amount of time and therefore demonstrates the most power.

In simplest terms, power is determined by two factors, movement speed and muscle force. Power can be improved by increasing one's movement speed, by increasing one's muscle force, or both. Movement speed is best improved by high quality skill training. Muscle force is best improved by high intensity strength training. Both power components are important for optimal athletic performance, and both must be practiced separately for best results: skill training to develop movement speed and strength training to develop muscle force.

Consider how strength training can benefit a technical athletic skill such as driving a golf ball. The golfer can gain distance by swinging the club faster, but at some point control will be lost and accuracy will be sacrificed. The golfer can also gain distance by developing greater muscle force through a well-designed strength training program. In this manner, the golfer can improve his driving distance and maintain his striking accuracy because he does not have to alter his normal swing.

Although there are unsubstantiated myths to the contrary, increased muscle strength does not hinder movement speed or joint flexibility. In fact, proper strength training enhances joint flexibility by alternately stretching and stressing the muscles throughout a full range of motion.

Several years ago, athletes were advised to avoid strength training altogether. A few years ago, coaches encouraged athletes to perform specific strength exercises for the muscle groups most involved in their event. Although this was a step in the right direction, the resulting muscle imbalance was a predisposing factor in numerous overuse injuries. Today, most college and professional athletic teams employ strength coaches to design balanced strength training programs that produce strong athletes and reduce the risk of injury. Proper strength training is undoubtedly a major contributing factor to the outstanding athletic performances of our day.

IMPROVED METABOLIC FUNCTION

Strength training is a vigorous, calorie burning activity. During a high-intensity strength training session, one's heart rate, blood pressure, and metabolic rate increase sharply, as discussed in Chapter 5. Of course, this temporary elevation in energy consumption is experienced in other large muscle activities such as jogging, swimming, and cycling. Strength training is different, however, in that it influences one's resting metabolism as well as one's exercise metabolism.

Endurance training burns large numbers of calories, but one's metabolism returns to the resting level within a few hours after exercise. Because strength training typically increases the amount of muscle tissue, the metabolic effects are experienced at rest as well as during exercise. This is due to the fact that muscle requires a constant supply of energy to sustain cellular functions. The more muscle one develops, the more energy is necessary 24 hours per day for protein synthesis and tissue maintenance.

Consequently, strength training has a double effect on energy utilization. It produces a large increase in metabolic rate during the training session and a small increase in metabolic rate throughout the day. For this reason, strength training is an excellent means for reducing body fat. Participants in the YMCA eight-week Weight Loss Program normally lose 8 pounds of scale weight. However, the average fat loss is 10 pounds and the average muscle gain is 2 pounds, for a 12-pound improvement in physical appearance.

Persons who like to eat should make a commitment to regular and progressive strength training. It is an efficient means of raising one's metabolic function, because muscle mass can be substantially increased and maintained through a 20-minute strength training program practiced three times per week.

REDUCED RISK OF INJURY

Perhaps the most important reason an active individual should perform strength training is to remain active and to avoid common injuries. Since World War II, progressive strength training has been the preferred method of injury rehabilitation. It is now understood that proper strength training is equally useful as a means of injury prevention. One reason there are relatively few neck injuries in football is the heavy emphasis coaches place on neck strengthening exercises.

A strong musculo-skeletal system offers some protection against injuries, but a balanced musculo-skeletal system is even more effective. While some athletic injuries are caused by collisions, most are simply the result of overtraining one muscle group and undertraining its counterpart. For example, distance runners frequently encounter injuries to the knee joint. Part of the problem is that distance running overstresses the muscles in the back of the legs and understresses the muscles in the front of the legs. This creates a front-to-back muscle imbalance that reduces the integrity of the knee joint and predisposes it to injury.

Although solutions are seldom simple, a first step to improve this situation is balanced strength training for all of the leg muscles. When all of the leg muscles are strong, there is considerably less chance of one muscle group overpowering another and causing an overuse injury.

Of course, it is also advisable for distance runners to strengthen their midsection and upper body muscles. Repetitive running places much stress on the lower back, so a strong midsection (front, back, and sides) is helpful for reducing low back injuries. Runners are not usually concerned about upper body strength, but these muscles are powerfully involved in the latter stages of a race and should also be strengthened in a balanced manner.

Running is not unique. Every athletic event involves some muscle groups more than others, and carries a certain risk of injury. Therefore, athletes should consider strength training for the purpose of preventing injuries as well as for the purpose of improving performance.

Athletes are not the only people who encounter muscle imbalance injuries. The business woman who sits at her desk from nine to five o'clock and the policeman who rides all day in his cruiser place much more stress on their low back muscles than on their abdominal muscles. As a result, many sedentary adults experience serious low back problems. In fact, low back discomfort is the most frequently cited reason for missed work days in the United States. Because 85 percent of low back problems are muscular in nature, strength training is generally beneficial from a preventive perspective.

It is emphasized that proper strength training can improve muscle balance and decrease the risk of injury. Conversely, improper strength training can be the cause of injury. Chapter 6 will present eight important guidelines for designing a safe and effective strength training program.

REACHING ONE'S STRENGTH POTENTIAL

Contrary to advertisements in popular muscle magazines, few persons who practice strength training will develop championship physiques, because the capacity to attain unusual muscle size is largely determined by genetic factors. However, almost everyone can look better, feel better, and function better as a result of intelligent strength training.

There are three keys to an efficient and effective strength training experience. They are: (1) muscle isolation, (2) stress intensification, and (3) personal motivation. Muscle isolation means training one muscle group at a time. Stress intensification means training with near maximum resistance. Personal motivation means training hard and is probably the single most important aspect of a successful strength training program.

The following chapters will provide detailed information to help the reader understand and implement these basic strength training concepts. Recommendations for exercise selection, exercise frequency, exercise duration, exercise intensity, exercise speed, exercise range, exercise progression, and exercise continuity are presented in light of recent research findings, along with practical advice on designing a personal strength training program.

As illustrated in Figures 1–1 and 1–2, the human body consists of several muscle groups, all of which have a specific role in movement mechanics. The purpose of this book is to challenge the reader to train sensibly and to reach maximum strength potential.

Strength training is an excellent activity for people who value physi-

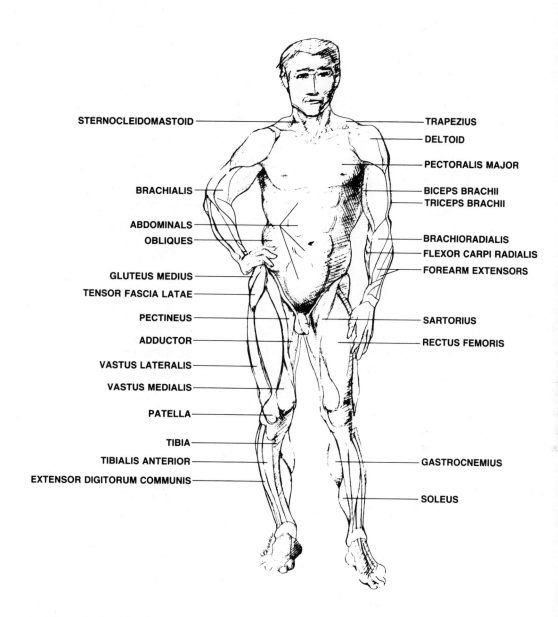

STERNOCLEIDOMASTOID

TRAPEZIUS

DELTOID

PECTORALIS MAJOR

BRACHIALIS

BICEPS BRACHII
TRICEPS BRACHII

ABDOMINALS
OBLIQUES

BRACHIORADIALIS
FLEXOR CARPI RADIALIS
FOREARM EXTENSORS

GLUTEUS MEDIUS
TENSOR FASCIA LATAE

PECTINEUS

SARTORIUS

ADDUCTOR

RECTUS FEMORIS

VASTUS LATERALIS
VASTUS MEDIALIS

PATELLA

TIBIA
TIBIALIS ANTERIOR

GASTROCNEMIUS

EXTENSOR DIGITORUM COMMUNIS

SOLEUS

Figure 1–1.   Muscles of the Body: Front

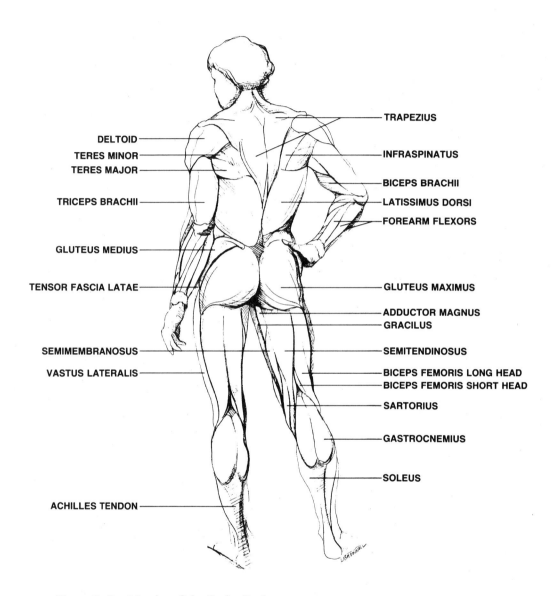

Figure 1-2.   Muscles of the Body: Back

cal fitness and personal appearance. Proper strength training demonstrates, perhaps better than any other activity, the positive relationship between physical exercise and physiological improvement. Anyone who is interested in physical fitness should set aside 60–90 minutes per week for regular and progressive strength training.

Chapter Two

Physiology of Strength Development

MUSCLE STRUCTURE

Muscle structure begins with two basic components, thick protein strands called myosin filaments, and thin protein strands called actin filaments. Small projections called cross-bridges extend from the myosin filaments to connect them to the surrounding actin filaments. Figure 2–1 illustrates schematically the way these filaments are arranged in a functional contractile unit known as a sarcomere.

Adjacent sarcomeres form myofibrils, which are the principal threads running throughout the muscles. Groups of myofibrils are bound together by a membrane called sarcolemma to form individual muscle fibers. Muscle fibers, in turn, are bound together by a membrane called perimysium into bundles of fibers known as fasiculi. These bundles of fibers are enclosed by a connective tissue called epimysium and function together as a muscle, such as the biceps. The structural and functional components of skeletal muscle are shown in Figure 2–2.

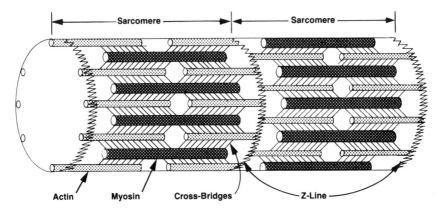

Figure 2–1. The smallest functional unit of muscle contraction, the sarcomere, consists of thin actin filaments, thick myosin filaments, and tiny cross-bridges which serve as coupling agents between the myosin proteins and the surrounding actin proteins.

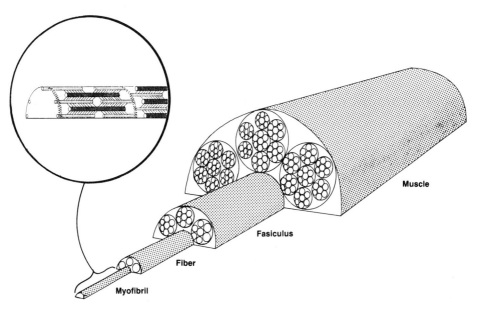

Figure 2–2. The structural and functional components of skeletal muscle.

MUSCLE PHYSIOLOGY

The most important components of skeletal muscle are the contractile proteins, actin and myosin. When activated, the thin actin filaments are pulled toward the center of the thick myosin filaments by the cross-bridges, which enables cross-linkages between the actin proteins and myosin proteins to occur.

The energy necessary for muscular movement is obtained from a rapid series of events beginning with nervous stimulation of the muscle cell. Upon receiving the nerve impulse, calcium ions are released from the sarcoplasmic reticulum, a system of tubules that has storage and distribution functions, which inactivates an inhibitory protein called troponin. When troponin is inactivated, myosin proteins function enzymatically to split adenosine triphosphate (ATP) into adenosine diphosphate (ADP) and energy. This ATP-splitting activity appears to take place at the cross-bridges and provides energy for the actin-myosin cross-linkages, which are responsible for muscular movement.

Upon cessation of nervous stimulation, the calcium ions are rebound to the sarcoplasmic reticulum, the inhibitory troponin proteins are reactivated, the enzymatic activity of the myosin proteins is prohibited, the ATP molecules are not split, energy is not released, cross-linkages do not occur, and the muscle relaxes.

MUSCLE CONTRACTION

When a muscle is activated, it produces tension and attempts to shorten. That is, it tends to pull its origin and insertion closer together. It should be understood, however, that muscle contraction actually means muscle tension and does not necessarily imply a change in muscle length. A contracting muscle may actually shorten, lengthen, or remain the same size.

Concentric Contraction. When a barbell is pressed from one's chest during the bench press exercise, the chest and triceps muscles exert force, shorten, and overcome the weightload. Whenever a muscle exerts force, shortens, and overcomes a resistance, it is said to contract concentrically. Concentric contractions are essential for overcoming the force of gravity and for enabling the exerciser to perform lifting movements.

Eccentric Contraction. When a barbell is lowered to one's chest during the bench press exercise, the chest and triceps muscles exert force, lengthen, and are overcome by the weightload. Whenever a muscle exerts force, lengthens, and is overcome by a resistance, it is said to contract eccentrically. It should be noted that if the chest and triceps muscles did not exert force during the lowering phase of the bench press exercise, the bar would drop onto the chest with the full force of gravity and cause considerable harm to the lifter. Eccentric contractions are, therefore, important for attenuating the force of gravity and for enabling the exerciser to perform safe, controlled lowering movements.

Isometric Contraction. If a barbell is momentarily held six inches above the chest during the bench press exercise, the chest and triceps muscles exert force, but do not change in length. They neither overcome the weightload nor are they overcome by the weightload. When a muscle exerts force, but does not change in length, it is said to contract isometrically. In other words, the force exerted by the muscle is equal to the force exerted by the resistance, and no movement occurs. Isometric contractions are important for stabilizing movements and for maintaining given joint positions.

Prime Mover Muscles

In any given joint action, the muscle that contracts concentrically to accomplish the movement is termed the prime mover. The prime mover, then, is the muscle that is principally responsible for the movement. For example, the biceps muscles are principally responsible for elbow flexion, and are, therefore, the prime mover muscle group for elbow flexion exercises, such as barbell curls (see Chapter 8). Many exercise movements involve more than one prime mover muscle group. Pull-ups, for example, require both shoulder extension and elbow flexion (see Chapter 8). In this case, both the latissimus muscles principally responsible for shoulder extension, and the biceps muscles principally responsible for elbow flexion, are prime mover groups.

Antagonistic Muscles

The muscle that produces the opposite joint action to that of the prime mover is called the antagonist. Because they extend the elbow, the triceps muscles are the antagonist to the biceps muscles. On the other hand, the triceps are prime mover muscles for elbow extension exercises such as triceps press-downs (see Chapter 8). For smooth elbow flexion, the triceps (antagonist muscles) must relax and lengthen as the biceps (prime mover muscles) contract and shorten. Conversely, for smooth elbow extension, the biceps (antagonist muscles) must relax and lengthen as the triceps (prime mover muscles) contract and shorten.

Stabilizer Muscles

For the desired movements to occur in certain joints, other joints must be stabilized. For example, to perform a standing barbell curl, the hips, back, and shoulders must be held in a stable position. Otherwise, instead of the barbell being curled to the shoulder, the shoulder girdle might be bent forward to the barbell. A similar situation occurs when performing push-ups. The midsection muscles must contract isometrically to maintain the body in a rigid position, thereby enabling one to exercise the chest and triceps muscles through a greater range of motion on each repetition. Muscles that perform this joint stabilizing function act as stabilizer muscles.

MUSCLE FORCE

Muscle contraction is the development of tension (force) within the muscle. Through a series of complex electrical and chemical changes, energy (ATP) is released, cross-linkages occur between the actin and myosin filaments, and both ends of the sarcomere are pulled toward the center. In the case of a concentric contraction, the muscle shortens, overcomes the external resistance, and accomplishes positive work. As the adjacent sarcomeres contract synchronously, the ends of the muscle move toward each other and produce the characteristic bulge schematically illustrated in Figure 2−3.

Motor Unit

Muscle contraction is regulated by the motor unit. A motor unit is made up of a single motor neuron and all the muscle fibers that receive stimulation from that nerve (see Figure 2−4). In large muscles, such as the rectus femoris, a single motor neuron may innervate several hundred

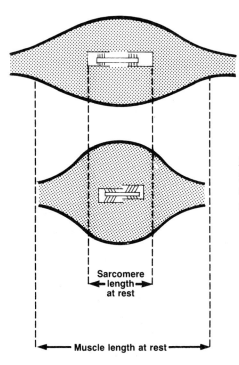

Sarcomere
←**length**→
at rest

←————— **Muscle length at rest** —————→

Figure 2-3. Changes in length of individual sarcomeres and entire muscle during concentric muscle contraction.

muscle fibers. In smaller muscles that produce precise movements, such as the muscles that move the eyes, each motor neuron innervates only a few muscle fibers.

Motor unit recruitment is the key to smooth, forceful, and sustained muscle contraction. Because the muscle fibers in a given motor unit are distributed throughout the muscle, only a few motor units need to be activated for coordinated muscle contraction. This arrangement allows individual motor units to alternately fire and rest when work is performed at submaximal strength levels.

Force Regulation

Because muscles are required to exert varying degrees of force (e.g., placing a light bulb in an overhead socket versus pressing a 90-pound barbell), some type of regulatory system is essential. There are two factors that affect the strength of a muscle contraction. These are the frequency of nerve impulses and the number of motor units activated. Fine adjust-

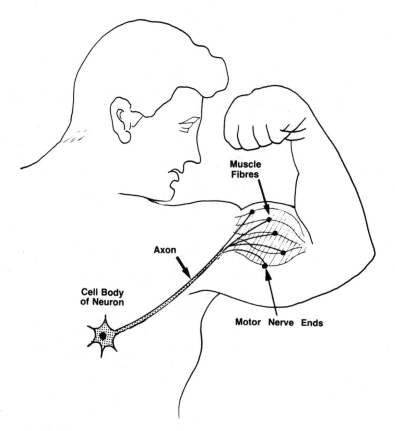

Figure 2-4. The motor unit consists of a single motor nerve and all of the muscle fibers that it innervates.

ments in muscle tension are produced by changes in the frequency of nerve impulses to the muscle fibers. As the frequency of nerve impulses increases, the strength of contraction increases; and as the frequency of nerve impulses decreases, the strength of contraction decreases. Gross variations in muscle tension are dependent upon the number of motor units activated by the central nervous system. The more units recruited, the stronger the contraction and vice versa. Under normal circumstances, different motor units fire independently. When maximum strength is required, nervous impulses may arrive more synchronously to enable the muscle fibers to produce maximum tension.

FIBER TYPES

Although the strength of contraction in skeletal muscles is primarily regulated by the central nervous system, the individual muscle fibers possess different contractile capacities. Individual muscle fibers may have fast-twitch characteristics or slow-twitch characteristics.

Slow-twitch muscle fibers bear the major burden in activities that require submaximal force production. These fibers are better suited for aerobic energy utilization because they contain more mitochondria, more endurance enzymes, more blood capillaries, and more intracellular fat. The slow-twitch fibers are able to produce low force contractions for a relatively long period of time. Elite distance runners may have up to 75 percent slow-twitch fibers in their leg muscles.

Fast-twitch muscle fibers bear the major burden in activities that require maximal force production. MacDougall (1985a) has reported larger cross-sectional areas, more contractile protein, and greater training-induced hypertrophy in fast-twitch muscle fibers. These fibers are better suited for anaerobic energy utilization because they have more myosin ATPase activity and more enzymes for anaerobic breakdown of glycogen and glucose. The fast-twitch fibers are able to produce high force contractions for a relatively short period of time. Olympic sprinters and jumpers may have up to 75 percent fast-twitch fibers in their leg muscles.

Research indicates that both muscle fiber types are actively recruited during maximal force production regardless of the movement speed. Research also shows that endurance training facilitates aerobic energy utilization in both slow-twitch fibers and fast-twitch fibers. However, there is no evidence that slow-twitch fibers can be turned into fast-twitch fibers or vice versa, since this would require changing the entire nerve innervation network.

Because strength events depend on anaerobic energy production, the person who is genetically endowed with a high percentage of fast-twitch muscle fibers may be more successful at weight training than the person who has a low percentage of fast-twitch muscle fibers.

Fiber Arrangement

Another factor that influences the strength of contraction is the muscle fiber arrangement. There are basically two types of fiber patterns, fusiform and penniform. Fusiform muscles have long fibers that run parallel to the line of pull. Muscles of this type produce little force but

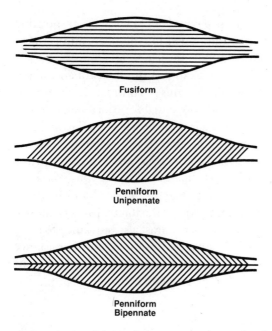

Fusiform

**Penniform
Unipennate**

**Penniform
Bipennate**

Figure 2–5. Schematic representations of a fusiform muscle, a unipennate muscle, and a bipennate muscle.

have a large range of movement. The biceps femoris muscle of the hamstrings group is fusiform. Penniform muscles have short fibers that run diagonally to the line of pull. Penniform muscles, therefore, produce greater force but have a smaller range of movement. Figure 2–5 presents schematic drawings of a fusiform muscle and two types of penniform muscles, penniform unipennate and the stronger penniform bipennate. The semitendinosus muscle of the hamstrings group is penniform uni-pennate, and the rectus femoris muscle of the quadriceps is penniform bipennate.

MUSCLE RELAXATION

The natural state of skeletal muscle is called relaxation. It is recalled that skeletal muscle contracts only upon nervous stimulation to do so. In the absence of such stimulation, the contractile mechanism is inactive, and muscle tension is not developed. Nonetheless, in a conditioned muscle, a firmness persists even when the muscle is relaxed. This is apparently due to the inherent characteristics of conditioned muscle fibers and connective tissue and is generally referred to as muscle tone.

An important aspect of muscle relaxation is the ability of an antagonistic muscle to relax when a prime mover muscle contracts. This process is known as reciprocal innervation and is essential for coordinated movements. At the same time that the prime mover muscle is cued to contract and shorten, the antagonistic muscle is cued to relax and lengthen. Actually, the degree of tension in each of the opposing muscle groups (prime movers and antagonists) is precisely regulated by the nervous system to enable smooth movements with varying degrees of speed and force.

Muscle relaxation is also essential to joint flexibility. Just as a muscle must be trained to contract more forcefully, it must also be trained to relax more completely. When a muscle is stretched to the point of resistance then maintained in that position for several seconds, it will adjust to its new length, relax, and allow itself to be stretched further.

MUSCLE FUNCTION

The function of skeletal muscle is to produce tension (force) that is generally translated into movement. Muscles are attached to bones by connective tissue called tendons. Tendons are actually extensions of the perimysium and epimysium, which enclose the muscle fibers and fiber bundles respectively. As illustrated in Figure 2–6, a skeletal muscle is attached between two bones. Contraction of the muscle produces force, which can move one bone through a range of degrees toward the other bone. The bone that remains stationary is considered the origin of the muscle, and the bone that moves is referred to as the insertion.

Joint Movements

The focus of this book is movement about the major joints of the human body. More specifically, exercises that, when properly applied, can increase the muscular force of the following joint movements will be presented. The joint movements are illustrated schematically in Figure 2–7.

> *Elbow Flexion:* Decreasing the angle between the lower arm and the
> upper arm.

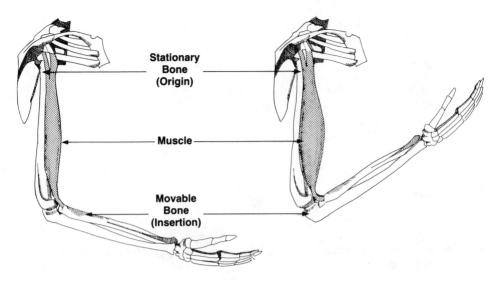

Figure 2-6. Contraction of a muscle resulting in the movement of one bone toward another. The stationary bone is referred to as the muscle origin, and the movable bone as the muscle insertion.

Elbow Extension: Increasing the angle between the lower arm and the upper arm.

Knee Flexion: Decreasing the angle between the lower leg and the upper leg.

Knee Extension: Increasing the angle between the lower leg and the upper leg.

Shoulder Adduction: Decreasing the angle between the upper arm and the side (downward-sideward movement).

Shoulder Abduction: Increasing the angle between the upper arm and the side (upward-sideward movement).

Shoulder Flexion: Increasing the angle between the upper arm and the chest (upward-forward movement).

Shoulder Extension: Decreasing the angle between the upper arm and the chest (downward-backward movement).

Shoulder Horizontal Flexion: Decreasing the angle between the upper arm and the chest (forward movement with the arms at right angles to the chest).

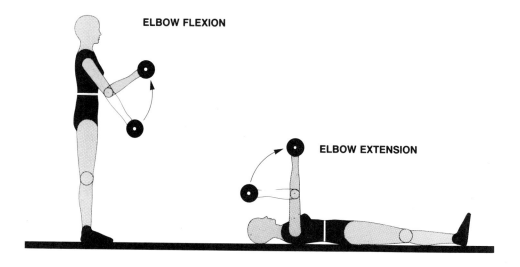

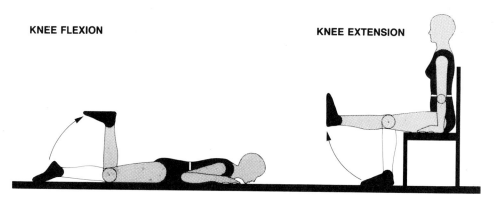

Figure 2-7. Schematic illustrations of joint movements.

Shoulder Horizontal Extension: Increasing the angle between the upper arm and the chest (backward movement with the arms at right angles to the chest).

Hip Flexion: Decreasing the angle between the thighs and the torso.

Hip Extension: Increasing the angle between the thighs and the torso.

Trunk Flexion: Decreasing the angle between the chest and the stomach.

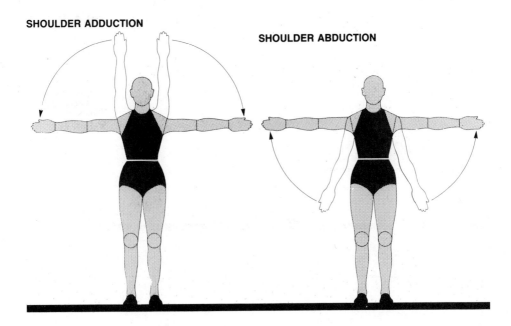

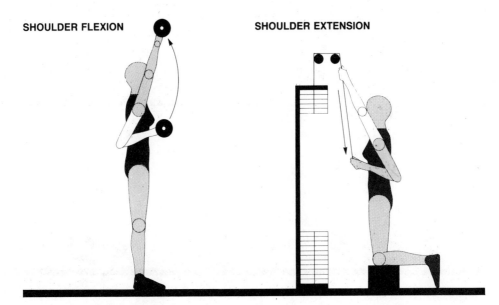

Figure 2–7. (continued)

SHOULDER HORIZONTAL FLEXION   **SHOULDER HORIZONTAL EXTENSION**

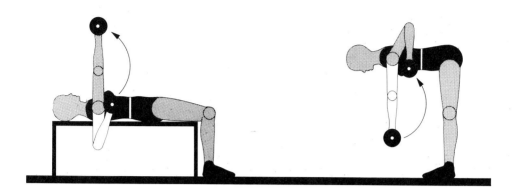

HIP FLEXION

HIP EXTENSION

TRUNK FLEXION

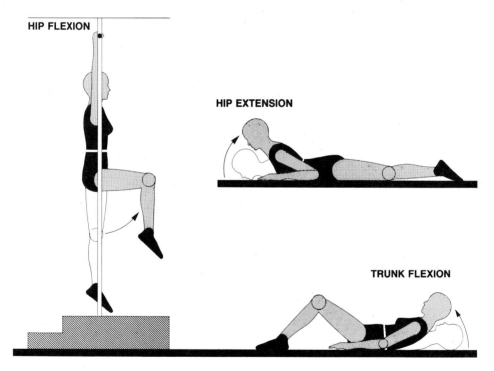

Figure 2-7.   *(continued)*

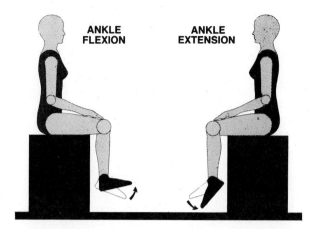
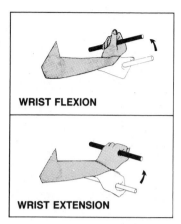

Figure 2–7. *(continued)*

Ankle Flexion: Decreasing the angle between the foot and the shin.

Ankle Extension: Increasing the angle between the foot and the shin.

Wrist Flexion: Decreasing the angle between the palm and the underside of the forearm.

Wrist Extension: Increasing the angle between the palm and the underside of the forearm.

Chapter Three

Factors That Affect Strength Performance

There are several factors besides the physiological properties of muscle tissue that influence one's effective muscular strength. These include biomechanical factors, lever arrangements, size factors, sex factors, and age factors. With the exception of cross-sectional size, which can be increased through strength training, these are factors over which we have no control. It is important to understand how each of these factors affects one's strength potential, because such knowledge helps the exerciser focus on personal improvement and individualized training.

BIOMECHANICAL FACTORS

It is quite possible for two persons who have developed the same amount of muscle tension to differ significantly in the amount of weight they can lift, because human movement is dependent upon a system of levers involving the long bones, joints, and muscles. The long bones act as levers, the joints serve as axes of rotation, and the skeletal muscles produce forces of sufficient magnitude to overcome resistance and cause movement.

Figure 3–1 illustrates a lever arrangement that is common in the human body. The biceps muscle operates as a third-class lever with respect to elbow flexion because the movement force is between the axis of rotation and the resistance. The distance between the axis of rotation (elbow) and the force (biceps insertion) is called the force arm, and the distance between the axis of rotation and the resistance (dumbbell) is called the resistance arm. The product of the resistance times the resis-

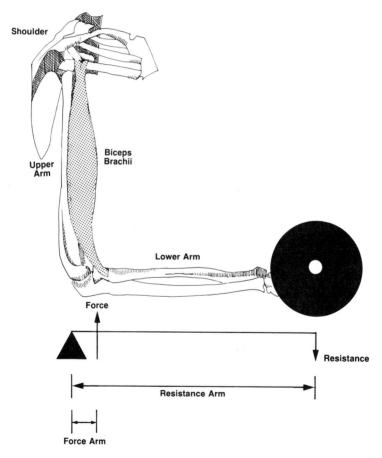

Figure 3–1. The biceps muscle operates as a third-class lever during elbow flexion. The movement force is between the axis of rotation and the resistance.

tance arm is equal to the product of the force times the force arm. Therefore, to determine how heavy a dumbbell one can hold at 90 degrees elbow flexion, one must multiply the muscular force by the force arm and divide the product by the resistance arm.

Example

John has a 12-inch forearm with a biceps insertion 1½ inches from the elbow joint. If John can produce 200 pounds of force in his biceps muscle, how heavy a dumbbell can he hold at 90 degrees elbow flexion? (Disregard the weight of his forearm.)

$$\text{Muscle Force} \times \text{Force Arm} = \text{Resistance} \times \text{Resistance Arm}$$

$$\frac{\text{Muscle Force} \times \text{Force Arm}}{\text{Resistance Arm}} = \text{Resistance}$$

$$\frac{200 \text{ Pounds} \times 1.5 \text{ Inches}}{12 \text{ Inches}} = 25 \text{ Pounds}$$

John's maximum biceps contraction of 200 pounds of muscle tension could hold a 25 pound dumbbell at 90 degrees elbow flexion.

This hypothetical example demonstrates that human lever systems require relatively large amounts of muscle force to overcome relatively small amounts of resistive force. Although this creates a mechanical disadvantage in movement force, it enables high rates of movement speed, which are vital to most athletic activities.

While progressive and systematic strength training is the key to developing muscle strength and hypertrophy, it should be understood that certain biomechanical factors affect one's ability to lift heavy weights. Consequently, one should not become discouraged if one trains as hard as a friend but cannot perform as well with heavier weights. The friend may simply have a built-in mechanical advantage.

Example

Bob also has a 12-inch forearm, but his biceps insertion is 2 inches from the elbow joint. If Bob can produce 200 pounds of force in his biceps muscle, how heavy a dumbbell can he hold at 90 degrees elbow flexion? (Disregard the weight of his forearm.)

$$\text{Muscle Force} \times \text{Force Arm} = \text{Resistance} \times \text{Resistance Arm}$$

$$\frac{\text{Muscle Force} \times \text{Force Arm}}{\text{Resistance Arm}} = \text{Resistance}$$

$$\frac{200 \text{ Pounds} \times 2.0 \text{ Inches}}{12 \text{ Inches}} = 33.3 \text{ Pounds}$$

Bob's maximum biceps tension of 200 pounds is equal to John's. However, due to a biceps insertion that is more favorable with respect to movement force, Bob can hold 33 percent more weight (33.3 pounds versus 25 pounds) at 90 degrees elbow flexion.

This example illustrates that certain inherited factors can profoundly influence one's effective muscular strength. It is therefore important to avoid comparisons with other persons and to focus on individual improvement regardless of the progress, or lack of progress, that others experience.

Third-Class Levers. Levers are classified according to the location of the axis of rotation, the resistive force, and the movement force. In a lever of the third class, the movement force is applied between the axis of rotation and the resistance, as shown in Figure 3−2. Because the biceps muscle inserts between the elbow joint (axis of rotation) and the hand (place where resistance is applied), it acts as a third-class lever. Most of the skeletal muscles function as third-class levers. As previously indicated, third-class levers favor movement speed over movement force.

Second-Class Levers. Levers of the second class place the resistance between the axis of rotation and the movement force (see Figure 3−2). This arrangement provides great movement force but is uncommon in the human body. One of the few examples of a second-class lever is opening one's mouth when chewing taffy or some other substance that resists pulling the teeth apart.

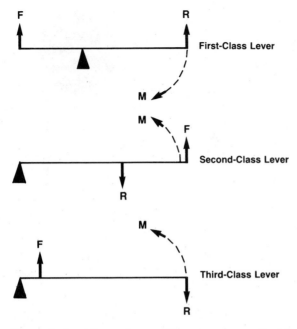

Figure 3—2. Three classes of levers as determined by the arrangement of the movement force (F), the resistance (R), and the axis of rotation. The resultant rotational movement is indicated by a broken line (M).

First-Class Levers. In first-class levers, the axis of rotation is between the movement force and the resistance, causing the ends of the lever to move in opposite directions (see Figure 3—2). The first-class lever arrangements found in the human body are similar to third-class lever arrangements in that they provide excellent movement speed at the expense of movement force. The triceps muscle is an example of a first-class lever because the elbow joint (axis of rotation) is between the muscle insertion and the hand (place where resistance is applied) as illustrated in Figure 3—3.

SIZE FACTORS

While it is true that biomechanical factors have an influence on one's ability to lift heavy weights, the contractile strength of a muscle is most closely related to its cross-sectional size. For example, the triceps muscle

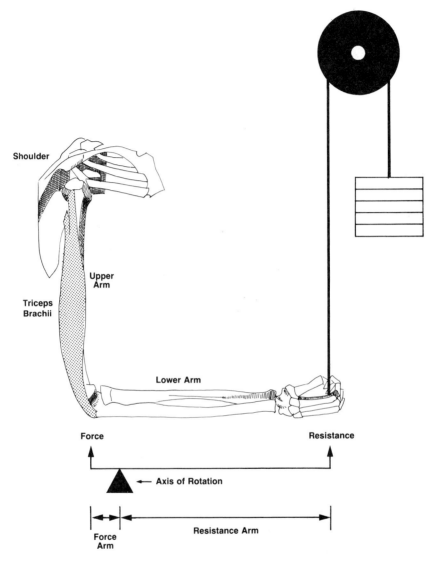

Figure 3-3. The triceps muscle operates as a first-class lever during elbow extension, because the axis of rotation is between the movement force and the resistance.

can produce approximately 2.88 pounds of force per square centimeter of cross-sectional area. It stands to reason, therefore, that the larger the cross-sectional area, the greater total force the triceps muscle can exert.

The cross-sectional area of one's muscle is initially determined by heredity, and a large-framed individual is likely to have larger muscles than a small-framed person. However, strength training can increase the cross-sectional size of a muscle by adding contractile proteins, actin, and myosin. Because there is little evidence that strength training can increase the total number of muscle fibers in humans, physiologists agree that greater muscle size results from the enlargement, not proliferation, of individual muscle fibers (Westcott, 1985g; MacDougall, 1985b). The increase in cross-sectional size of a muscle as a result of strength training is called hypertrophy. Conversely, the decrease in muscle size that occurs when training is discontinued is known as atrophy.

The length of the muscle belly may also be an important factor with respect to muscle size (see Figure 3−4). The muscle belly represents the

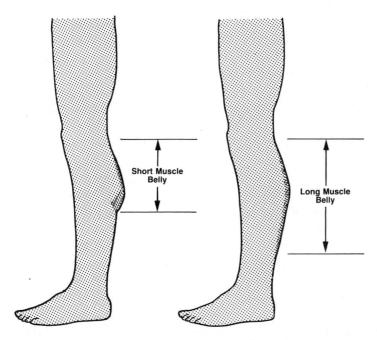

Figure 3−4. Comparison of a short-belly and long-belly gastrocnemius muscle. The length of the muscle belly may affect the potential size and strength of a muscle.

actual muscle length between the tendon attachments. Other things being equal, it is assumed that the person with a longer muscle belly has the potential to develop greater muscle size and strength than the person with a shorter muscle belly. The length of the muscle belly appears to be an inherited characteristic that cannot be changed through training. Most people have a mixture of long-bellied muscles, medium-bellied muscles, and short-bellied muscles. Those rare individuals who possess a large percentage of long-bellied muscles are most likely to be successful in weightlifting and physique competition.

SEX FACTORS

Women who engage in strength training programs develop muscular strength at about the same rate as men. Research by Westcott (1974, 1976, 1979) indicates that both males and females can increase the strength of their bench press muscles (chest, anterior shoulders, and triceps) by 3 to 6 percent per week, depending on age factors and the training program utilized. It is also known that males and females do not differ in strength per square centimeter of muscle tissue. However, with respect to muscle size and effective muscle strength, there are definite sex-related differences. Although males and females gain strength at similar rates, postpubescent males begin with larger muscles, which provides a significant strength advantage. Furthermore, strength training increases muscle size to a far greater degree in males than in females. The reason appears to be related to the male sex hormone, testosterone, which plays a major role in muscle growth and hypertrophy.

By virtue of their genetic make-up, males have a greater potential for muscle size and strength than females. Nonetheless, most females can develop pound-for-pound muscle strength that compares favorably to that of their male counterparts. Westcott (1986i) evaluated 900 adults on a Nautilus Leg Extension Machine. The average male performed 10 repetitions with 62 percent of his bodyweight, and the average female performed 10 repetitions with 55 percent of her bodyweight. Figures 3–5 and 3–6 illustrate the strength development of a typical college-aged male and college-aged female over a five-week training period utilizing the bench press exercise. As shown in Figure 3–5, the male subject increased his bench press by 20 pounds during the training period, and the female subject increased her bench press by 10 pounds. When examined in terms of percentage improvement, however, both subjects gained

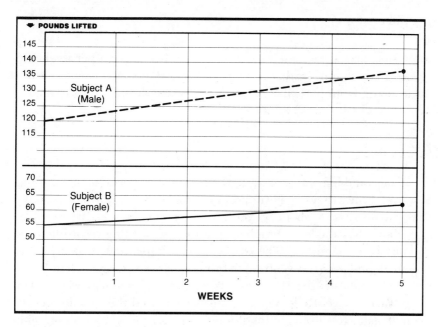

Figure 3−5. Increase in bench press strength as indicated by actual amount of weight lifted. (Bodyweights: male = 160 lbs., female = 95 lbs.)

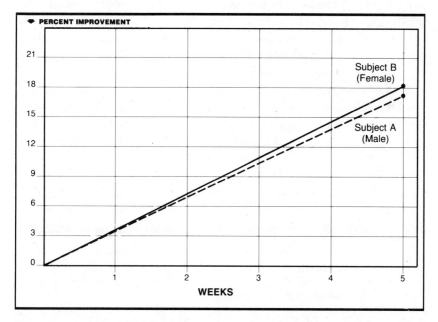

Figure 3−6. Increase in bench press strength as indicated by percent improvement. (Bodyweights: male = 160 lbs., female = 95 lbs.)

strength at about the same rate, approximately 4 percent per week (see Figure 3−6). It appears that females may obtain the same strength bene-fits as males from participation in similar strength training programs.

AGE FACTORS

Males and females gain strength through the process of maturation. However, unless they engage in strength training activities, their strength begins to decrease at about age 30. This phenomenon is not irreversible, as evidenced by the large number of older weightlifting record holders and physique champions. The key to strength improvement at any age is systematic and progressive strength training. However, research by West-cott (1979) indicates that the rate of strength development may be related to age factors (see Table 3−1). Westcott compared the average weekly strength gains for three groups of female subjects (N = 14) training with the bench press exercise. One group consisted of young girls under 13.5 years of age. On the average, the girls in this group increased their strength by 6.4 percent per week, which is an exceptionally high rate of strength gain. A second group was composed of older girls between 13.5 and 19 years of age. The average strength improvement for the girls in this group was 4.7 percent per week. The third group was made up of young women over the age of 19, and the average strength gain in this group was 2.6 percent per week.

These data suggest that strength may be developed more rapidly in younger females than in older females. It should be noted that the women over 19 years of age improved their strength by almost 3 percent per week, a rate that compared favorably to that reported for college males

Table 3−1   Rates of Strength Development for Female Subjects of Different Ages

Age Group	Average Strength Increase Percent per Week
9−13.5 years	6.4
13.5−19 years	4.7
19−27 years	2.6

training with the bench press exercise (Westcott, 1974). The higher rates of strength development observed in the younger females are very interesting. Research by Micheli (1983) indicates that preadolescent males respond in a similar manner to systematic strength training. Apparently, strength training is more effective during periods of physical growth and maturation.

The author has found no reason to restrict young children from strength training activities. Clarke's (1971) longitudinal study of boys in Medford, Oregon, revealed a consistent ratio of strength to size during 10 years of growth (ages 8–18). Empirical evidence suggests that young children are generally more capable of handling their bodyweight (e.g., climbing trees, ropes, flagpoles) than are adolescents or adults. For those children who are not strong enough to lift their bodyweight, it is far more beneficial to curl a barbell 10 times than to struggle with a single pull-up. Both the physical strain and the mental trauma that accompany unsuccessful attempts at bodyweight exercises are unnecessary and can be avoided through proper strength training activities. Perhaps the greatest advantage of weight training over bodyweight exercises is that the resistance can be accommodated to the strength of each individual, regardless of size, sex, or age.

TRAINING EXPERIENCE

Training experience implies the length of time one has been involved in a strength training program. Generally speaking, the person who has trained regularly for two years will make smaller strength gains than the person who has trained for only two weeks. During the early stages of a strength training program, improvement usually comes quickly; but as people get closer to their genetic potential, strength increases are much smaller and less frequent. In fact, progress appears to slow considerably during the first three months of training (Westcott, 1985a, 1985c). Figure 3–7 illustrates a typical strength improvement curve over a three-month training period. Although the participant achieves a 40 percent strength gain during the first month, the strength increase is only 10 percent during the second month, and about 2.5 percent during the third month.

The process of expending more and more effort and experiencing less and less improvement can be discouraging. It is therefore important to use training experience in the most productive manner possible. First,

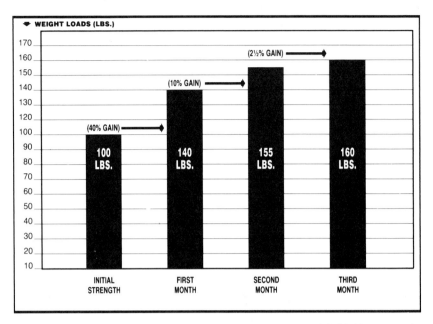

WEIGHT LOADS (LBS.)

Figure 3–7. Sample 3-month improvement for athlete with initial leg extension weightload of 100 lbs.

it must be understood that if one continues to do the same exercise, progress will plateau after several weeks. Second, due to the motor learning and skill specificity aspects of muscular activity, a change in exercise is usually accompanied by a higher rate of performance improvement.

Consequently, experienced strength trainers should routinely alter their training program in order to observe progress and maintain motivation. For example, Bill has been unable to complete more than 10 repetitions with 150 pounds in the leg extension exercise. Rather than remain on a plateau in this exercise, he replaces leg extensions with leg presses. By so doing, he continues to train the quadriceps muscles, but the movement pattern is different enough to require a new neuromuscular response pattern. The result is noticeable performance improvement in the leg press exercise due to both learning factors (see Chapter 5) and muscle development. When progress in the leg press plateaus, Bill should return to the leg extension exercise. Within a few training sessions he should exceed his previous performance level in this exercise.

In summary, experienced strength training participants are less likely to see regular progress because they are closer to their strength potential. By frequently changing exercises, they can continue to make performance improvements, which stimulates strength development and enhances training motivation.

TRAINING TECHNIQUE

Technique has a profound but paradoxical influence on one's response to strength training. In effect, poor training technique is associated with a higher rate of performance improvement but a lower rate of strength gain. That is, by training in a fast, momentum-assisted manner one can hoist heavier weightloads. However, because more momentum means less muscle tension, the performance increases are much greater than the strength increases.

Actually, poor form always violates the principle of muscle isolation by incorporating assisting muscle groups to initiate the lifting movements. For example, Tom can cheat curl 150 pounds by bending forward and using his large trunk extensor muscles to start the barbell moving upward. Unfortunately, the biceps muscles are only partially involved in this impressive-looking exercise. Once the trunk extensors overcome the barbell's inertia, momentum plays the major role in completing the lifting movement.

On the other hand, slow training technique facilitates muscle isolation and stress intensification. Because slow movements reduce the momentum factor, less weight can be lifted. However, the target muscle groups are fully responsible for lifting and lowering the weightload. As a result, they produce more muscle tension and receive greater stimulus for strength development.

For example, Tom can curl only 75 pounds in strict form because the biceps are not helped by larger muscle groups. While the weightload may not be as impressive, Tom places greater stress on the biceps muscles this way than in the momentum-assisted cheat curl.

High intensity exercise does not necessarily imply heavy training weightloads. How the training weightload is lifted has much greater bearing on one's strength development.

In summary, poor training technique enables heavier weightloads, but typically produces smaller strength gains due to the offsetting influence of assisting muscle groups and momentum. Strict lifting form requires lighter weightloads but emphasizes muscle isolation and stress intensification, thereby resulting in greater strength improvement.

TRAINING SPECIFICITY

People frequently equate hard work with success, but this is only true when there is a strong relationship between the work being done and the desired outcomes. Both a 10-mile run and 3 sets of heavy squats are hard work, but the physiological responses to each type of exercise are quite different. Both the serious distance runner and the serious weight-lifter train an hour or more each day, but their physical appearances are strikingly dissimilar. Training that involves long periods of low intensity exercise may develop cardiovascular endurance but does not improve muscle strength. Conversely, training that involves short periods of high intensity exercise develops muscle strength but may not improve cardiovascular endurance. Experiments with laboratory animals (Gordon, 1967) indicate that endurance training produces an increase in endurance enzymes, but a decrease in contractile proteins, and that strength training produces an increase in contractile proteins, but a decrease in endurance enzymes.

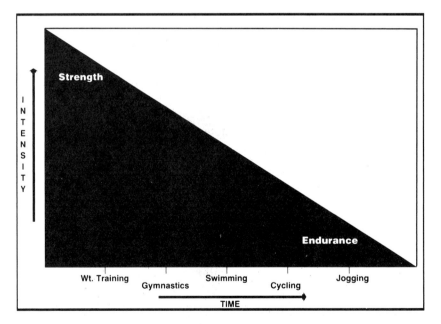

Figure 3-8. Position of various activities along the strength-endurance continuum. Note that strength-related activities are of relatively high intensity and short duration.

One should probably train in a specific manner to obtain specific results: strength training for muscle development and endurance training for cardiovascular development. Figure 3–8 indicates the approximate positions of various activities along the strength-endurance continuum. Note that strength-related activities are of relatively high intensity and short duration, whereas endurance-related activities are of relatively low intensity and long duration.

ALARM

One occasionally reads of an incredible feat of strength, such as a mother lifting a car off a child pinned beneath it. Such incidents suggest that each of us possesses greater strength than we ordinarily use or even realize we have. Apparently, certain mechanisms within the neuromuscular system prevent the muscles from producing the maximum force possible except under conditions of alarm, thereby protecting the muscles and connective tissues from possible injury. Strength coaches who are aware of this phenomenon sometimes shout at an athlete during a lifting attempt in order to reduce these built-in inhibitions and trigger more powerful muscle contractions. Perhaps more important, Ikai and Steinhaus (1961) have indicated that one of the effects of progressive strength training is a resetting of the neuromuscular inhibition level, which permits the athletes to voluntarily use a greater percentage of their maximum strength. In other words, well-trained individuals may be capable of using some of their reserve strength under normal training conditions.

MUSCLE STRETCH

One of the factors that influences the strength of a muscle contraction is the initial length of the muscle fibers. A muscle produces greater tension when it is stretched just prior to contraction. Ask a friend to perform a standing long-jump. Notice that the thigh muscles are momentarily placed on stretch by a quick-sitting movement just before they contract powerfully and propel the body several feet through space. Similar prestretching movements can be observed in the leg, torso, and shoulder muscles of shot putters as they impart force to the 16-pound ball. Likewise, when one stretches the chest muscles immediately before beginning the upward phase of the bench press exercise, considerably more force can be exerted. Although the mechanisms that enable a muscle to generate greater force upon being stretched are not fully understood, it would appear that both the elastic properties of muscle tissue and the alignment of the actin and myosin filaments are major contributing factors.

Chapter Four

Principles of
Strength Training

People participate in strength training programs for many reasons, but predominant among these is a desire for larger and stronger muscles. Although the degree of muscular attainment is influenced by certain inherited factors such as somatotype, limb length, muscle length, angle of tendon insertion, and percentage of fast-twitch and slow-twitch muscle fibers, most people can achieve marked increases in muscle strength and hypertrophy through a systematic and progressive program of weight training. Research indicates that proper training produces the following adaptations within the muscular system: a higher concentration of contractile proteins, a greater number of myofibrils per muscle fiber, a greater number of capillaries per muscle fiber, an increased amount of connective tissue, a larger percentage of muscle fibers available for force production, and more efficient energy utilization.

There is no question that people who have engaged in widely varying programs of strength training have experienced muscular gains. Promoters of particular systems of strength augmentation are quick to point out how many champions their programs have developed. Far less publicized is the fact that strict adherence to many of these training regimens often results in muscle injury, strength decrement, and discouragement. The truth is, regardless of the training program one follows, the probability of experiencing desirable training consequences is closely related to the number of basic training principles observed by the exerciser. Conversely, the probability of encountering undesirable training consequences is closely related to the number of basic training principles violated by the exerciser.

A well-designed strength training program should incorporate the following fundamental principles of muscle development to insure gradual improvement in strength and to reduce the risk of tissue injury: Principle of Stress Adaptation, Principle of Rebuilding Time, Principle of Near-Maximum Resistance, Principle of Controlled Movement Speed, Principle of Full-Range Movements, Principle of Muscle Balance, and Principle of Training Specificity. While it is not the purpose of this chapter to compare different systems of muscle training, one rather unusual program will be presented to illustrate certain principles of muscle development that contribute to optimal training effectiveness.

It is reported that in ancient Greece, Milo of Crotona initiated an Olympic Games by carrying a full-grown bull across the stadium. The training program that Milo used to accomplish this incredible feat of strength was very simple. Every day, beginning with the day the bull was born, he lifted the bull onto his shoulders and ran across the barnyard. While not the most sophisticated method of strength augmentation, Milo's training program satisfied some of the principles of muscle development and apparently led to the achievement of his training objective.

PRINCIPLE OF STRESS ADAPTATION

When a muscle is stressed beyond its normal demands, it reacts in some way to that stress. If the stress is slightly greater than normal, the muscle responds positively and becomes stronger. That is, after a temporary decrease in ability following the training session, the muscle gradually rebuilds to a higher level of strength. On the other hand, if the imposed stress is too great, the muscle reacts negatively and tissue damage results. For instance, if one hoes the garden for 5 minutes on Monday, 10 minutes on Tuesday, 15 minutes on Wednesday, and so on, the hands will gradually become calloused and hoeing can be continued for long periods of time without skin discomfort. However, if one begins by hoeing the garden for 2 hours on Monday, blisters are likely to develop and hoeing will have to be discontinued for several days until the skin heals. The phenomenon that occurs beneath the skin is actually quite similar. The person who progressively increases the intensity and duration of gardening activity will gradually condition the muscles involved, but the person who does too much too soon will experience muscle deconditioning during the several days required for the repair of damaged tissues.

The muscles respond to the stress of a strength training session in the same manner. If the intensity of the workout is increased gradually, the muscles respond positively and gain strength. However, if the intensity of the workout is increased abruptly, the muscles react negatively and tissue damage may occur.

Example

Milo of Crotona trained his muscles in strict accordance with the Stress Adaptation Principle. Each day that Milo went to the barnyard he found his prize bull slightly heavier than the day before. These small, daily increments in weightload provided an ideal training stimulus for Milo's muscles, namely gradual and progressive stress adaptation. It is important to note that Milo did not pick up a baby bull one day and a yearling the next day. Instead, he demonstrated a patient and controlled approach to strength training, which is the most effective way to promote injury-free muscle development.

Application

Strength training must be progressive. As soon as the muscle can accommodate a particular resistance, slightly greater stress should be applied to stimulate further strength improvement. Perhaps more important, large increments in resistance should be avoided. At best, disrespect for this training principle may result in chronic muscle fatigue and lack of progress. At worst, too much stress too soon may cause injury to muscle or connective tissue. Many people work as close to the breaking point as possible in an attempt to obtain their strength goals more quickly. Playing the edge may facilitate faster strength gains, but it is just as likely to cause injury and frustration. It is better to set long-range goals and experience gradual improvement than to seek overnight results and spend several weeks rehabilitating injuries. Determining when to increase the training load is not really difficult. Each new workout should provide a clear indication as to whether the current weightload is too heavy, too light, or just about right. Observing a simple rule of not increasing the resistance of any exercise by more than 5 percent per week should insure sensible and safe progression.

PRINCIPLE OF REBUILDING TIME

When a muscle is stressed beyond its normal demands, a certain amount of time is required for the tissues to recover and make positive physiological adaptations. If the time between workouts is too short, the muscle is unable to rebuild to a higher level of strength before being stressed again. The cumulative effects of insufficient rebuilding time are chronically fatigued muscles that actually decrease in strength. Conversely, if the non-training interval is too long, the muscle will gradually return to its original level of contractile force.

Because the length of the rest interval depends on the intensity of the work interval, more hours are required for muscle rebuilding following a hard workout than after an easy workout. Each person must experimentally determine the optimal recovery period between workouts for his or her particular training program. Figure 4−1 schematically illustrates that the contractile force of a muscle decreases during a training session due to the stress imposed on it, but increases to a slightly higher strength level during a recovery period of sufficient duration.

As indicated in Figure 4−2 when too little rest is obtained between training sessions, the muscle is unable to rebuild to a higher level of strength prior to the next workout. The cumulative stress of repeated training sessions without sufficient time for muscle rebuilding leads to chronic training fatigue, and the muscles actually become weaker rather than stronger.

When too much rest is taken between successive workouts, the muscle initially rebuilds to a higher level of strength, but gradually returns to its original strength level prior to the next training session. Because the new strength level is not maintained indefinitely, it is important that the subsequent training stimulus occur near the peak of the

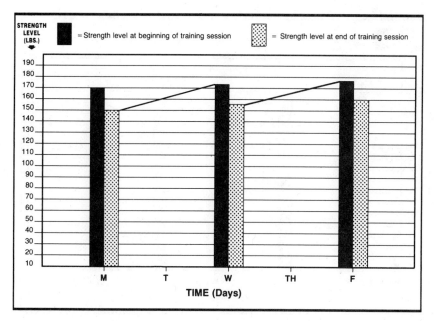

Figure 4–1. Hypothetical pattern of muscle response when recovery period is appropriate with respect to training intensity. When sufficient rest is obtained between training sessions, the muscle rebuilds to a slightly higher level of strength.

rebuilding curve. Taking too much rest between training sessions may not be harmful, but the lack of strength gains can be frustrating. The consequences of an extended recovery period are illustrated schematically in Figure 4–3.

Example

It is reported that Milo of Crotona performed only one training task per day, that of hoisting the bull onto his shoulders and running across the barnyard. We may also assume that Milo, a member of the privileged society, did not engage in other exhausting work that would interfere with his recovery processes. Under these training conditions, Milo's 24-hour rest period was apparently adequate to permit positive adaptation and muscle rebuilding.

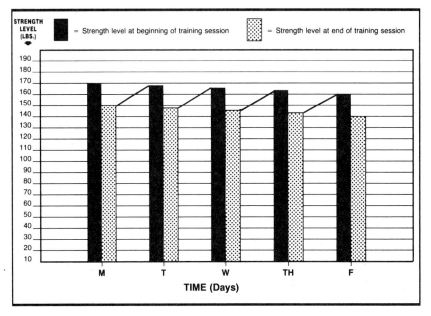

Figure 4−2. Hypothetical pattern of muscle response when recovery period is too short with respect to training intensity. When too little rest is obtained between training sessions, the muscle is unable to rebuild to a higher level of strength.

Application

Strength training programs must insure sufficient rebuilding time between workout sessions to enable the muscles to attain higher strength levels. A decrease in performance generally indicates a need for more rest rather than a need for more work. Almost without exception, persons who begin a strength training program are eager to attain their goals and set out to do so in a hurry. Unfortunately, these good intentions often result in insufficient rest between workouts, which prohibits full recovery and maintains the muscles in a fatigued state. In addition to being a source of discouragement, fatigued muscles are highly susceptible to injury, particularly when worked harder in an attempt to force improvement.

Research findings indicate a direct relationship between the duration of the training session and the duration of the recovery

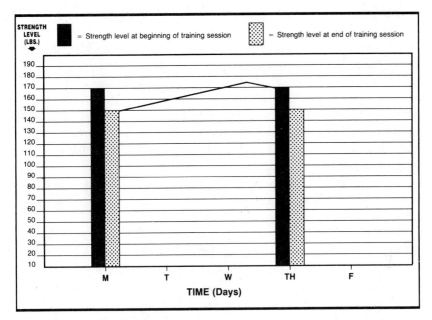

STRENGTH LEVEL (LBS.)

■ = Strength level at beginning of training session

▦ = Strength level at end of training session

190
180
170
160
150
140
130
120
110
100
90
80
70
60
50
40
30
20
10

M   T   W   TH   F

TIME (Days)

Figure 4–3. Hypothetical pattern of muscle response when recovery period is too long with respect to training intensity. When too much rest is taken between training sessions, the muscle initially rebuilds to a slightly higher level of strength, but gradually returns to its original strength level.

period. As discussed in Chapter 5, Westcott (1974) studied the relationship between the length of the training session and the length of the rebuilding period. Although all of the training groups experienced substantial strength gains, the subjects who performed short and more frequent workouts seemed to obtain better results than the subjects who endured long and less frequent workouts.

The optimal length of the recovery period for a particular training program must be determined individually through trial and error procedures. However, one should realize that increasing the difficulty of the workout routine may require a corresponding adjustment in rebuilding time to insure continued strength improvement. If successive workouts fail to produce strength gains, one should consider a longer rebuilding period.

PRINCIPLE OF NEAR-MAXIMUM RESISTANCE

There are basically two ways to apply stress to one's muscles. One may perform numerous repetitions against low resistance (e.g., jogging, cycling, rope jumping, calisthenics) to improve cardiovascular endurance, or one may perform few repetitions against high resistance (e.g., lifting heavy weights) to improve muscular strength. Each type of training stimulus produces specific results. If one's objective is to develop muscular strength and hypertrophy, the training program should focus on few repetitions with heavy resistance.

Weight training authorities generally agree that weightloads around 75 percent of maximum are highly effective for promoting strength gains.

Regardless of one's maximum weightload in a given exercise, the 10RM (10 repetition maximum) weightload usually corresponds to about 75 percent of that maximum. In other words, the heaviest weightload that can be lifted 10 times is approximately 75 percent of the maximum weightload that can be lifted one time.

Persons who train with 10RM weightloads apply sufficient muscular stress to produce strength improvement. Weightloads less than 65 percent of maximum are not as useful for strength augmentation, while weightloads greater than 85 percent of maximum may increase the risk of injury.

The Principle of Near-Maximum Resistance is often referred to as the "overload" principle because strength gains are dependent upon weightloads over and above those routinely encountered in one's daily activities. Because a true muscle overload would prevent the muscle from contracting concentrically, "near-maximum resistance" is a more accurate description of this training phenomenon.

Example

By performing a single lift with a heavy resistance (the bull), Milo insured that his muscles would be subjected to an adequate training stimulus for strength development. However, Milo was probably playing too close to the edge for comfort. Executing a single lift with maximal resistance is more appropriate for demonstrating strength than for building strength. Using the heaviest resistance possible for every workout is a dangerous practice, particularly when the weightload is wearing horns.

Application

The recommended number of repetitions for promoting optimum gains in strength varies from individual to individual. Most people obtain good results by training between 65 percent (15 repetitions) and 85 percent (5 repetitions) of maximum weightload (Berger 1962b, 1962c). Better results may be realized when training with 70 percent (12 repetitions) to 80 percent (8 repetitions) of maximum weightload (Westcott, 1986j).

PRINCIPLE OF CONTROLLED MOVEMENT SPEED

When training with weights, it is important to raise and lower the weightload in a slow and controlled manner to insure consistent application of force throughout the exercise movement. Such a movement subjects the muscles to a more or less steady stress during both the lifting phase (concentric contraction) and the lowering phase (eccentric contraction). Experiments with force plates have revealed that lifting movements performed at a moderate speed require a relatively even application of muscular force. On the other hand, executing fast repetitions with a barbell or dumbbell is equivalent to throwing the weight. It seems that fast movements demand excessive muscular force at the beginning of the lift, but practically no muscle force is necessary during the midrange of the lift. Tests have demonstrated that during explosive lifting movements, the exerciser is actually lifted by the weights. In fact, electronic traces of a quick press with a 60-pound barbell show a range of forces from over 100 pounds at the start of the lift to less than zero during the middle part of the lift. There can be little doubt that rapidly accelerating or decelerating a weightload subjects the muscles to widely varying levels of stress. Consequently, this type of training is less likely to improve muscle strength and more likely to cause tissue injury.

It should also be recalled that intensity is the key to strength development. As the speed of movement increases, however, the weightload must necessarily be reduced unless assisting muscles are utilized. Consequently, weightloads that are light enough to permit rapid movements are less effective for promoting strength gains. One can train with light loads and fast repetitions or with heavy loads and slow repetitions, but the person interested in developing muscular strength is advised to use the latter method. Controlled lifting and lowering movements with relatively heavy weightloads are basic to safe and effective strength training programs.

Example

It is assumed that Milo treated his prize bull carefully, neither throwing the bull overhead nor dropping him abruptly to the ground. By lifting and lowering the bull in a slow, controlled manner, Milo prevented injury to both himself and the bull. He also provided his muscles with a greater stimulus for strength development.

Application

Weightlifting movements should be performed with a steady application of force. This applies to both the lowering phase and the lifting phase because the same muscles are involved in both movements. Fast movements are by no means recommended for improving muscular strength. If the exercise can be performed rapidly, the exerciser is using too little resistance or too many assisting muscle groups to initiate the movements. Generally speaking, the lifting movement (concentric contraction) should take about 2 seconds and the lowering movement (eccentric contraction) should take about twice as long, approximately 4 seconds. In other words, a set of 10 repetitions should be completed in about 60 seconds.

PRINCIPLE OF FULL-RANGE MOVEMENTS

When a muscle is exercised through a full range of motion there is little chance of decreasing joint flexibility. However, when opposing muscle groups are not exercised, or when partial movements are performed, there is a possibility of restricting one's range of joint mobility. For instance, it is not uncommon for a person desiring to bulk up the biceps to perform "cheat" curls in such a way that the arms remain partially flexed throughout the exercise. Such a practice could eventually lead to larger, shorter biceps muscles which might hinder full elbow extension. This undesirable outcome would be even more probable if the exerciser did not execute full-range movements for the antagonistic muscle group, the triceps.

Full-range movements also provide the muscles with a greater training stimulus, because the distance over which a muscle moves a weight-load is proportional to the amount of work done:

Work = Force × Distance

Consequently, the muscle that moves a weightload over a complete range of motion performs more work than the muscle that executes a partial movement with the same weightload. Full-range movements are, therefore, beneficial in terms of both flexibility development and strength development. Finally, since most athletic skills require application of force over the maximum distance possible (e.g., throwing, striking, kicking), performing less than full-range exercise movements has limited practical value.

Example

Assuming that Milo performed his daily exercise task by squatting beneath the bull, placing the bull squarely on his shoulders, and gradually rising to an erect position, he probably achieved full range of motion in his knee extensor muscles. It is doubtful, however, that he exercised his hip extensor muscles or back extensor muscles through a full range of motion. Lack of strength and flexibility in these muscle groups is often a contributing factor to lower back pain. Milo's training program was highly specific and geared toward attaining a rather unusual objective. However, if he had understood the importance of full-range movements, he might have performed some supplemental training exercises to maintain his flexibility and facilitate his strength development.

Application

Whenever possible, one should select exercises that incorporate a full movement range. Also, exercises for opposing muscle groups should be paired to assure joint flexibility. For example, when the biceps muscles are fully contracted, the opposing triceps muscles are fully extended, and vice-versa. If complete muscle contraction cannot be achieved, the resistance is probably too heavy and should be reduced. It is almost always better to execute full-range movements with appropriate resistance than to perform partial movements with excessive resistance.

PRINCIPLE OF MUSCLE BALANCE

Weight training programs should be designed to promote strength development in all of the major muscle groups. Emphasizing certain muscle groups can produce muscle imbalance which may, in time, lead to muscle injury. Too often, athletes and weightlifters perform strengthening exercises only for the muscles that are prime movers in their particular event or activity. For example, sprinters and jumpers typically perform several strengthening exercises for their quadriceps muscles but few, if any, strengthening exercises for their hamstring muscles. This often results in an overpowering quadriceps group and a relatively weak hamstrings group that becomes highly susceptible to injury. The same problem is encountered by throwers who deliberately strengthen their triceps muscles but ignore their biceps, and by competitive powerlifters who execute numerous sets of bench presses, incline presses, and other chest strengthening exercises without performing corresponding exercises for their back muscles.

Whenever a muscle group is disproportionately stronger than its antagonist, the latter is predisposed to injury. This is not to say that paired muscle groups should be trained to exactly equal strength. For example, the quadriceps muscles are stronger than the hamstring muscles at the knee joint (knee extension vs. knee flexion), but the hamstring muscles are stronger than the quadriceps muscles at the hip joint (hip extension vs. hip flexion). Consequently, one would normally use more resistance in knee extension than knee flexion and in hip extension than hip flexion.

The important point is that the muscle groups should not be trained in isolation. If the muscles on one side of a joint are worked, then the muscles on the opposite side of the joint should likewise be worked, even though the workloads may not be identical.

The problem of maintaining desirable muscle balance can be simplified by training all of the major muscle groups (see Chapter 6). This requires one exercise for each of the following muscle groups: quadriceps, hamstrings, hip adductors, hip abductors, low back, abdominals, chest, upper back, shoulders, biceps, triceps, neck flexors, and neck extensors. Furthermore, one should not work the wrist extensors without also training the wrist flexors or the calf muscles apart from the shin muscles.

The Principle of Muscle Balance is a necessary counterpart to the Principle of Training Specificity. To many people, training specificity means training only those muscle groups that are prime movers for a particular event. For example, a thrower may perform a variety of triceps exercises to improve his shot put performance. However, unless the triceps exercises are balanced with biceps exercises, the athlete will increase the risk of overuse injuries. It appears that overly specialized training has been at least partially responsible for numerous injuries to muscle and connective tissue. The extra time and effort necessary to train one's muscles in a comprehensive and balanced manner seems to provide substantial dividends in terms of injury prevention and overall muscular development.

Example

Since Milo both lifted the bull up and set the bull down, he exercised most of his major muscle groups, right? No, the same muscles were used concentrically during the lifting phase and eccentrically during the lowering phase. That is, by increasing the number and rate of motor units firing in the quadriceps muscles, Milo was able to gradually extend his knees and lift the bull off the ground. Conversely, by decreasing the number and rate of motor units firing in the quadriceps muscles, Milo was able to gradually flex his knees and lower the bull gently back to earth. It is important to note that it was the gradual increase and decrease of muscle tension in the quadriceps that allowed Milo to both lift and lower the bull. The force of gravity is all that is needed to lower the weightload. Therefore, the same muscles that contract concentrically to lift the weightload must act eccentrically to keep the weightload from dropping too quickly and causing injury.

This being the case, Milo apparently violated the principle of muscle balance. Unless he also performed exercises for the opposing muscle groups, he developed strength disproportionately and may have experienced pains and problems not recounted in the traditional story.

Application

Regardless of specific training objectives, one should include exercises for all of the major muscle groups when designing a training program. Symmetrical and proportionate development of one's musculature sets a firm foundation for further strength improvement and minimizes the risk of injury to muscle and connective tissue.

Maintaining relative balance between opposing muscle groups is particularly important for preventing injuries. It is noted that the predisposing factor in a large percentage of hamstring injuries is muscle imbalance between a relatively strong quadriceps group and a relatively weak hamstrings group. By training all of the major muscle groups in pairs, many such injuries can be avoided and the quality of athletic performance can be enhanced.

PRINCIPLE OF TRAINING SPECIFICITY

Training specificity means different things to different people. Some people believe that we should train one way to develop muscle strength and another way to develop muscle endurance. Others believe that we should train one way to increase muscle strength and another way to increase muscle size. Some people recommend one type of training to gain weight and another type of training to lose weight. Many coaches feel that athletes should train one way for one sport and another way for another sport.

In reality, strength training provides a stimulus to increase the amount of contractile proteins within a muscle. This increases muscle density, which results in greater muscle strength, greater muscle weight, greater muscle size, greater muscle tone, and greater caloric requirements. Because there is a direct relationship between the weight that can be lifted one time and the weight that can be lifted fifteen times, an increase in muscle strength produces a corresponding increase in muscle endurance.

While it is true that different sports emphasize different muscle groups, athletes should develop overall muscle strength to maintain muscle balance and to reduce the risk of injury. As discussed in the previous section, training only the prime mover muscle groups can be counterproductive.

It is recommended that the Principle of Training Specificity be applied to energy systems rather than to muscle groups. For example, sprinters should spend the majority of their training time performing high intensity, anaerobic exercise. Conversely, distance runners should spend the majority of their training time performing low intensity, aerobic exercise.

It is also suggested that the Principle of Training Specificity be applied to sports skills rather than to muscle groups. For example, a high jumper should strengthen all of the major muscle groups to enhance power production. However, it is necessary to repeatedly practice proper technique in order to achieve better performance. Because the high jump is a very complex athletic event, the majority of practice time should be spent executing full speed jumps at challenging heights.

It is not advisable to perform an athletic event with extra weight, or to imitate a sports skill with added resistance. To do so alters the neuromuscular pattern for the movement, and generally interferes with performance progress. For example, jumping with ankle weights requires a slightly different neuromuscular response than jumping without ankle weights. Therefore, any improvement in strength that may result from training with ankle weights is offset by undesirable changes in movement speed and technique. When the jumper removes the ankle weights for competition, the previous movement speed and smoothness is likely to be missing, and the performance will probably be poorer than expected.

Example

Milo practiced the specific skill of hoisting a bull overhead and running across the barnyard. By consistently performing this movement pattern, he undoubtedly developed a high level of neuromuscular efficiency. However, unless Milo performed complementary exercises, he violated the Principle of Muscle Balance and increased his risk of overuse injuries.

Application

Every strength training program should be specific with respect to the exerciser. That is, every individual should train in the manner that produces the best personal results. The Principle of Training Specificity should be applied to the appropriate energy system and to the desired performance technique. With regards to specific exercises, it is recommended that one exercise be performed for each of the major muscle groups. By combining the Principles of Muscle Balance and Training Specificity, the exerciser can achieve a higher level of performance with a lower risk of injury.

SUMMARY OF TRAINING PRINCIPLES

In the final analysis, there are three fundamental features of an effective program of strength development: muscle isolation, stress intensification, and personal motivation. Essentially, one singles out a specific muscle group and gradually applies greater and greater stress to it. There are three simple steps one should follow to train in this manner. First, one should identify a particular muscle group to be strengthened (e.g., triceps muscles). Second, one should select an exercise for which the target muscle group is a prime mover (e.g., triceps extensions). Third, the exerciser must progressively increase the intensity of the training stimulus (e.g., increase the weightload by 5 percent when 12 repetitions can be completed).

Given this basic framework for improving muscular strength, one should train in accordance with the Principles of Strength Development presented in this chapter. Adherence to these guidelines should increase the probability that muscle strength will be gained, that muscle balance will be maintained, and that muscle injury will be avoided.

The principles of Stress Adaptation, Rebuilding Time, Near-Maximum Resistance, Controlled Movement Speed, Full-Range Movements, Muscle Balance, and Training Specificity apply to all persons and all training programs. However, each individual should employ these principles in the manner that is most effective for promoting his or her own strength development. For example, some persons will increase strength more quickly than others, and some persons will recover more quickly than others. The important thing is that one's personal training program incorporates each of these training principles in a way that is compatible with his or her own physiological and psychological characteristics. "Know yourself and be yourself" is an excellent motto for successful strength training experiences.

Chapter Five

Research on Strength Training

During the past few years, the author has been privileged to conduct several research studies on strength training. This chapter will present the results of the following investigations:

1. Effects of different training frequencies on strength development.
2. Effects of different training sets on strength development.
3. Effects of different training repetitions on strength development.
4. Effects of different training speeds on strength development.
5. Effects of different training times on strength development.
6. Effects of strength training on blood pressure.
7. Effects of strength training on heart rate.
8. Effects of strength training on cardiovascular performance.
9. Effects of strength training on muscle performance.
10. Effects of strength training on body composition.

Much of the research on strength training is of a short-term nature. That is, most studies look at a particular training variable over a one- to three-month training period. As a rule, the training participants are college students or members of an athletic team. Most of the studies presented here were conducted with adult men and women who had no prior strength training experience. Consequently, the results tend to represent this segment of the population and may not accurately describe the training response of highly conditioned athletes. For the most part, these research findings are generalizable to persons who are beginning a strength training program. The following chapter, "Designing the Strength Training Program," will incorporate the research results into several recommendations for safe, effective, and efficient strength training.

EFFECTS OF DIFFERENT TRAINING FREQUENCIES ON STRENGTH DEVELOPMENT

Many people in our fast-paced society have difficulty maintaining a regular training schedule. While most strength training proponents advocate an every-other-day work-rest sequence, not everyone can follow this training pattern. Some enthusiasts find a few minutes every day for a short workout, while others endure a lengthy training session once or twice a week.

The purpose of Westcott's (1974) study was to compare different frequencies of training on strength development. In an attempt to isolate the frequency variable, total training workloads were equated on a weekly basis. More specifically, all 55 subjects performed 60 repetitions per week with the bench press exercise. Group one trained one day per week and completed all 60 repetitions (12 sets of 5 repetitions) in a single session. Group two trained two days per week, and completed 30 repetitions (6 sets of 5 repetitions) each session. Group three trained three days per week, and performed 20 repetitions (4 sets of 5 repetitions) each session. Group four trained five days per week, and executed 12 repetitions (2 sets of 6 repetitions) each session. Table 5–1 presents the training protocols followed by the four experimental groups.

All of the subjects were tested for maximum bench press strength (1 RM) at the beginning and every two-and-a-half weeks during the seven-and-a-half-week training period. As indicated in Table 5–1, groups three and four experienced higher rates of performance improvement than groups one and two. The frequent, short-duration workouts produced an average strength gain of 23 percent, and the infrequent, long-duration workouts produced an average strength gain of 18 percent. These results are illustrated graphically in Figure 5–1.

Table 5–1   Effects of Different Training Frequencies on the Development of Muscle Strength

Group	Repetitions per Training Session	Training Sessions per Week	Repetitions per Week	Mean Percent Increase
One	60	1	60	19%
Two	30	2	60	16%
Three	20	3	60	24%
Four	12	5	60	21%

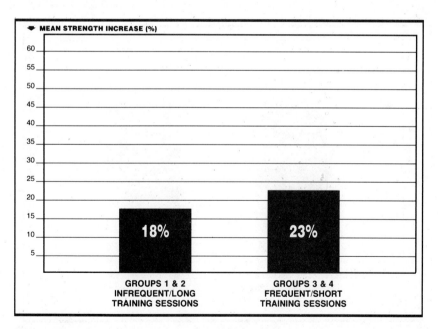

Figure 5–1.   Comparison of Strength Gains from Infrequent/Long Training Sessions and Frequent/Short Training Sessions.

Another study by Westcott (1986e) compared two strength training sessions per week with three strength training sessions per week. Group two performed 11 Nautilus exercises on Mondays and Thursdays, and group three performed 11 Nautilus exercises on Mondays, Wednesdays, and Fridays. After eight weeks of training, both groups increased their strength by approximately 48 percent (see Figure 5–2).

Summary

Based on the findings of the first study, it would appear that frequent, short-duration training sessions are more effective than infrequent, long-duration training sessions for improving performance in the bench press exercise. Based on the findings of the second study, it would appear that two and three evenly spaced Nautilus training sessions per week are equally effective for developing muscle strength. As a general guideline, it is recommended that most participants follow a three-day-per-week strength training schedule. In the event of a missed workout, two training sessions per week should produce comparable strength gains.

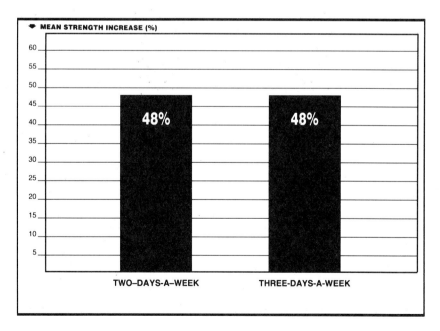

Figure 5–2. Comparison of Strength Gains from Two-Day-a-Week and Three-Day-a-Week Training Schedules.

EFFECTS OF DIFFERENT TRAINING SETS ON STRENGTH DEVELOPMENT

There is general confusion as to how many sets of a given exercise one should perform for best results. Bodybuilders typically execute multiple sets with each exercise, whereas most adult fitness centers advocate a single set training policy.

The DeLorme-Watkins Program

The concept of training with a certain number of sets and repetitions was introduced by Thomas DeLorme and Arthur Watkins in the late forties. Their work with muscle rehabilitation produced one of the first systematic and progressive weight training programs to receive approval from both medical and physical education professionals. Their original strength training routine consisted of three sets of 10 repetitions each. The first set of 10 repetitions is performed with 50 percent of the heaviest weightload that can be lifted 10 times and serves as a first-level warm-up. The second set of 10 repetitions is conducted with 75 percent of the heaviest weightload that can be lifted 10 times and serves as a second-level warm-up. The final set of 10 repetitions is executed with the heaviest weightload that can be lifted 10 times and is the actual stimulus for strength development. The heaviest weightload that can be lifted 10 times is called the 10 repetition maximum or 10RM weightload.

Example

The heaviest weightload that John can press 10 times in succession (10RM weightload) is 100 pounds. According to the DeLorme-Watkins training formula, John should do the following workout.

First Set: 10 repetitions with 50 pounds (50% 10RM weightload).

Second Set: 10 repetitions with 75 pounds (75% 10RM weightload).

Third Set: 10 repetitions with 100 pounds (100% 10RM weightload).

As John's muscles respond to the training stimulus he will be able to complete more than 10 repetitions with 100 pounds. DeLorme and Watkins recommended that a new 10RM weightload be established when the exerciser can perform 15 repetitions with the previous 10RM weightload. This ensures gradual and progressive loading of the muscles in accordance with the stress adaptation principle. This program represents what is generally known as a double progressive training approach, because the exerciser alternately increases the number of repetitions and the exercise weightload.

Although the actual process of strength development is influenced by a variety of factors (see Chapter 3), a typical response to the DeLorme-Watkins training program might resemble the hypothetical pattern of progression shown in Table 5−2. It should be noted that the DeLorme-Watkins approach incorporates an alternate day training schedule.

DeLorme and Watkins' program for strength development involves two warm-up sets and one set requiring maximum effort. The final set of 10 repetitions with the 10RM weightload provides the essential training stimulus for positive strength adaptations to occur. Beginning in 1962, Richard Berger began to experiment with different combinations of sets and repetitions in an attempt to determine the most effective training program for improving muscular strength.

The Berger Program

One of Berger's first experiments (1962b) dealt with the optimum number of repetitions one should perform when training with a single set. His findings indicated that one set of the 4RM, 6 RM, or 8RM weightload

Table 5−2 Hypothetical Pattern of Progression in the Bench Press Exercise Using the DeLorme-Watkins Training Program

Week	Monday	Wednesday	Friday
1	60 lbs. × 10	60 lbs. × 10	60 lbs. × 10
	90 lbs. × 10	90 lbs. × 10	90 lbs. × 10
	120 lbs. × 10	120 lbs. × 12	120 lbs. × 13
2	60 lbs. × 10	New 10RM	65 lbs. × 10
	90 lbs. × 10	found to be	97.5 lbs. × 10
	120 lbs. × 15	130 lbs.	130 lbs. × 10
3	65 lbs. × 10	65 lbs. × 10	65 lbs. × 10
	97.5 lbs. × 10	97.5 lbs. × 10	97.5 lbs. × 10
	130 lbs. × 11	130 lbs. × 11	130 lbs. × 12

produced greater strength gains than one set of the 2RM, 10RM, or 12 RM weightload. He therefore concluded that training with 3 to 9 repetitions encompassed the optimum number of repetitions for increasing strength when training with one set, three times weekly.

Because persons who train with free weights typically perform more than one set of an exercise, Berger conducted several studies involving various combinations of sets and repetitions. His best-known study (1962a) compared all combinations of one, two, and three sets with 2, 6, and 10 repetitions per set. The results of this study suggested that three sets of 6 repetitions each with the 6RM weightload was the most effective training stimulus for gaining muscular strength. Although subsequent investigations by Berger (1963) and O'Shea (1966) did not confirm the superiority of this training program, three sets of 6 repetitions with the 6RM weightload has become a very popular training format, particularly for beginners and noncompetitive weight trainers.

When one begins training with the 6RM weightload, one will probably execute fewer than 6 repetitions in the second and third sets due to the cumulative effects of fatigue. However, as strength increases, the exerciser will be able to complete 6 repetitions in all three sets. At that time the weightload should be increased by 5 percent and the strength building process begun anew. Although strength development is a phenomenon influenced by a number of factors (see Chapter 3), a typical response to the Berger training program might resemble the hypothetical pattern of progression indicated in Table 5–3. Like the DeLorme-Watkins program, the Berger system utilizes a three-day-per-week training schedule.

Table 5–3 Hypothetical Pattern of Progression in the Bench Press Exercise Using the Berger Training Program

Week	Monday	Wednesday	Friday
1	100 lbs. × 6	100 lbs. × 6	100 lbs. × 6
	100 lbs. × 5	100 lbs. × 6	100 lbs. × 6
	100 lbs. × 4	100 lbs. × 4	100 lbs. × 6
2	105 lbs. × 6	105 lbs. × 6	105 lbs. × 6
	105 lbs. × 4	105 lbs. × 5	105 lbs. × 6
	105 lbs. × 3	105 lbs. × 4	105 lbs. × 4
3	105 lbs. × 6	110 lbs. × 6	110 lbs. × 6
	105 lbs. × 6	110 lbs. × 4	110 lbs. × 5
	105 lbs. × 6	110 lbs. × 4	110 lbs. × 5

However, unlike the single training stimulus provided by the final set in the DeLorme-Watkins system, Berger's program calls for maximum effort on all three sets, because each set of 6 repetitions is done with the 6RM weightload.

The Pyramid Program

In 1979, Westcott compared the training effects of the DeLorme-Watkins system and the Berger system, along with a third program that involved three sets with increasing weightloads and decreasing repetitions. The latter is a type of program commonly referred to as a pyramid system of training, because each set is done with more weight and fewer repetitions. The pyramid program was based on the exerciser's 1RM weightload, that is, the heaviest weightload that could be lifted one time. The first set consisted of 10 repetitions with 55 percent of the 1RM weightload, the second set required 5 repetitions with 75 percent of the 1RM weightload, and the third set was a single lift with 95 percent of the 1RM weightload.

Example

The heaviest weightload that Susan can bench press once (1RM weightload) is 100 pounds. According to Westcott's training formula, Susan would perform the following workout:

First Set: 10 repetitions with 55 pounds (55% 1RM weightload).

Second Set: 5 repetitions with 75 pounds (75% 1RM weightload).

Third Set: 1 repetition with 95 pounds (95% 1RM weightload).

The pyramid program is similar to the DeLorme-Watkins program in that both involve two progressively heavier warm-up sets and one set designed to produce the training effect. They are different with respect to the relative amount of resistance used for the training stimulus in the final set. The DeLorme-Watkins program requires 10 repetitions with a submaximum resistance (10RM weightload). The pyramid program requires 1 repetition with a near-maximum resistance (95 percent 1RM weightload).

Program Comparison

All of the participants in Westcott's study gained muscular strength, and the rates of strength development for the three training groups were quite similar. Comparative results of the Berger system, the DeLorme-Watkins system, and the pyramid program are summarized in Table 5−4.

While differences in the rate of strength improvement were not statistically significant, it is interesting to note two apparent trends with regard to these training programs. First, the training systems that required only one strenuous training set (DeLorme-Watkins program and pyramid program) seemed to be more effective than the system that incorporated three strenuous training sets (Berger program). Second, the training system based on the 1RM weightload (pyramid program) and the training system based on the 10RM weightload (DeLorme-Watkins program) appeared to be equally effective for increasing muscular strength.

The DeLorme-Watkins program requires a total of 30 repetitions, the Berger system a total of 18 repetitions, and the pyramid program a total of 16 repetitions. Yet, the results of Westcott's study indicate that the total number of repetitions may be a secondary consideration in terms of strength development. The more important factor seems to be near-maximum muscular effort with relatively heavy resistance. One repetition with 95 percent of the 1RM weightload (pyramid program), 6 repetitions with the 6RM weightload (Berger system), and 10 repetitions with

Table 5−4 Summary of Strength Gains Obtained with the DeLorme-Watkins, Berger, and Pyramid Training Programs

Training Group	Training Program	Mean Percent Strength Improvement per Week
Berger	6 × 6RM 6 × 6RM 6 × 6RM	3.7%
DeLorme-Watkins	10 × 50% 10 RM 10 × 75% 10RM 10 × 100% 10RM	4.3%
Pyramid	10 × 55% 1RM 5 × 75% 1RM 1 × 95% 1RM	4.3%

the 10RM weightload (DeLorme-Watkins program) all require near-maximum muscular effort and therefore produce a positive training effect. Another study by Berger (1965) indicated that it is not advisable to train with less than two-thirds of the 1RM weightload if one is interested in strength development, regardless of the number of repetitions performed. This is in agreement with the Principle of Near-Maximum Resistance (see Chapter 4).

It is interesting to note that the advantage of performing more than one set at maximum effort has never been clearly established. Both Theodore Hettinger, the physician who conducted numerous experiments on isometric strength training during the early sixties, and Ellington Darden, Director of Research for Nautilus Sports/Medical Industries, believe that one set per exercise at maximum effort is sufficient training stimulus to promote optimum strength development.

One-Set Versus Two-Set Strength Training

Advocates of Nautilus strength training insist that one set of 10 repetitions properly performed to the point of momentary muscle failure is the most effective way to increase muscle strength. Because most persons who train with weights perform three or more sets with each exercise, the author designed a research study to compare the effects of training with one, two, and three sets on Nautilus equipment (Westcott, 1986j). Due to injuries, illness, and dropouts, the number of subjects who completed the three-set program was too low to include in the data analyses. Consequently, the research study actually compared one-set strength training with two-set strength training.

The subjects, 28 women and 16 men, trained three times per week for a period of four weeks. Half of the subjects (14 women and 8 men) performed one set of 10 repetitions on each of the following Nautilus machines: (1) leg extension, (2) leg curl, (3) torso pullover, (4) arm extension, and (5) arm curl. The other subjects (14 women and 8 men) executed two sets of 10 repetitions on each of the Nautilus machines. All of the subjects were previously untrained and performed no other strength-related activities during the course of the study.

The results revealed no significant difference in strength gain between the subjects who performed one set of each exercise and the subjects who performed two sets of each exercise. As shown in Figure 5−3, the one-set training group made a 56 percent increase in strength

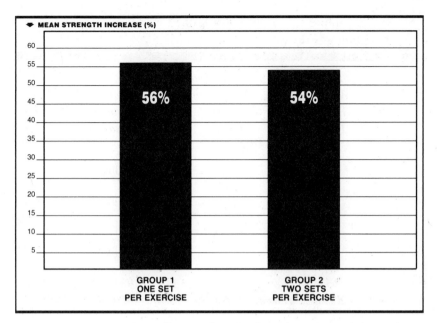

Figure 5–3. Comparison of Strength Gains from One-Set Training and Two-Set Training.

performance, and the two-set training group made a 54 percent increase in strength performance.

The data were also analyzed by sex. The men who trained with one set and the men who trained with two sets both experienced a 41 percent increase in strength. The women who trained with one set and the women who trained with two sets experienced strength gains of 76 percent and 70 percent, respectively. These results are presented in Table 5–5.

Because one set of 10 repetitions per exercise produced the same strength improvement as two sets of 10 repetitions per exercise, it would appear that single-set training is an effective and efficient means of developing muscle strength when using Nautilus machines. This finding tends to support recommendations for single-set Nautilus training programs made by Peterson (1982), Riley (1982), and Darden (1982).

Both the male and female subjects experienced significant improvement in muscle strength over the four-week training period. The greater percent increase in muscle strength attained by the women (70 percent strength gain versus 40 percent strength gain) was most likely due to their lower initial strength levels.

Table 5-5   Comparison of Strength Gains for One-Set Training and Two-Set Training by Sex

Group	Mean Initial Weightload (Sum of Five Exercises)	Mean Final Weightload (Sum of Five Exercises)	Mean Weightload Increase	Mean Percent Increase
Men One-Set	328 lbs.	462 lbs.	134 lbs.	41%
Men Two-Set	341 lbs.	480 lbs.	139 lbs.	41%
Women One-Set	135 lbs.	237 lbs.	102 lbs.	76%
Women Two-Set	155 lbs.	264 lbs.	109 lbs.	70%

As side notes, the mean bodyweight remained the same for all subjects. The mean increase in thigh circumference measured six inches above the knee cap was .4 inches for all subjects. The observed gain in muscle size without a gain in bodyweight suggests a change in body composition. Apparently, the increase in muscle was matched by a corresponding decrease in fat (Westcott, 1984a). This training phenomenon will be discussed in more detail later in the chapter.

Summary

Based on the research presented in this section, it would appear that the essential stimulus for strength improvement is a single exercise set with near-maximum resistance. One study showed no difference between single-set and multiple-set training for strength development. Because two of these studies demonstrated excellent strength results with a 10-repetition exercise set, this would seem to be a reasonable training guideline. From a safety perspective, performing one set with the 10RM weightload carries a lower risk of injury than training with heavier weightloads. The following section will take a closer look at the optimal number of training repetitions.

EFFECTS OF DIFFERENT TRAINING REPETITIONS ON STRENGTH DEVELOPMENT

There is an inverse relationship between the weightload utilized for a particular exercise and the number of repetitions that can be executed. When one uses the heaviest weightload possible, only a single lift can be performed. As the weightload is reduced, more repetitions can be completed.

Between 1948 and 1970, a considerable amount of research was conducted to determine the optimum number of repetitions for developing muscle strength with isotonic training. DeLorme and Watkins (1948) devised one of the first systematic approaches to progressive resistance exercise based on three sets of 10 repetitions with increasing weightloads.

Berger (1962a) compared nine different strength training programs involving all combinations of one, two, and three sets with 2, 6, and 10 repetitions and found that three sets of 6 repetitions produced the greatest strength gains. Berger (1962b) later reported the results of another study in which one set of 3−9 repetitions proved equally effective for strength improvement.

In a 1963 investigation, Berger found no significant differences among training programs utilizing 2, 6, or 10 repetitions per set. O'Shea (1966) also found no significant differences among training programs using 2 and 3 repetitions, 5 and 6 repetitions, or 9 and 10 repetitions. In a similar study, Withers (1970) found no significant differences among training programs incorporating 3, 5, or 7 repetitions per set.

During the seventies, Nautilus literature had a major impact on strength training protocols (Darden, 1977), and one set of 8−12 repetitions became standard procedure for most strength training participants. Many people experienced good results with 8−12 repetitions per set, and research on this training variable was largely discontinued.

Westcott conducted two studies comparing 8-repetition training and 12-repetition training. The subjects who trained with 8 repetitions used the heaviest weightload that could be performed 8 times, and the subjects who trained with 12 repetitions used the heaviest weightload that could be performed 12 times. The first study (1986j) showed no differences between the two training groups, but the second study (1986h) revealed better results with 8-repetition training.

Jones (1986) suggested that some individuals respond better to low-repetition training, while other individuals respond better to high-repetition training due to inherent physiological characteristics. He found that some subjects reached 75 percent of their initial strength level after 4 or 5 repetitons, while others required 15–16 repetitions to reduce their starting strength level by 25 percent. If Jones' hypothesis were correct, it might partly account for the inconsistent findings with regards to optimum training repetitions.

Westcott (1986f) examined differences in muscle performance with a given submaximum resistance. The 87 subjects, 49 men and 38 women, were tested on a Nautilus 10 degree chest machine to determine the heaviest weightload that they could perform one time. After a five-minute rest, the participants completed as many repetitions as possible with 75 percent of their maximum weightload.

The findings of this study revealed a wide range of repetitions with 75 percent of maximum weightload in the Nautilus 10 degree chest exercise. Two subjects completed only 5 repetitions, while one subject performed 24 repetitions with the same relative resistance (see Figure 5–4). As shown in Table 5–6, the mean score was 10.8 repetitions, with a standard deviation of 3.1. The male subjects had a mean score of 10.2 repetitions, and the female subjects had a mean score of 11.6 repetitions.

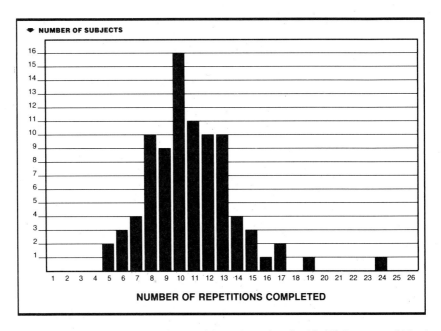

Figure 5–4. Distribution of Repetitions Completed with 75 Percent of Maximum Weightload.

Table 5-6 Descriptive Statistics for Repetitions Completed with 75 Percent of Maximum Weightload

Subjects	Repetitions		
	Range	*Mean*	*Standard Deviation*
Male	5-19	10.2	2.8
Female	6-24	11.6	3.2
All	5-24	10.8	3.1

Based on these results, it would appear that individuals vary considerably in the number of repetitions they can perform with 75 percent of maximum weightload. Stated differently, it would seem that there is considerable variation in the number of repetitions necessary to reduce one's starting strength level by 25 percent. The statistical analyses indicated that four out of six subjects experienced a 25 percent strength decrement between 8–14 repetitions. However, one out of six subjects required 7 or less repetitions, and one out of six subjects required 15 or more repetitions to reduce their initial strength level by 25 percent.

It would therefore appear that some people can perform more work with a given submaximum resistance due to greater muscle endurance. Because all of the subjects trained regularly with one set of 8–12 repetitions, it would also appear that this ability may be independent of the training procedures. These findings seem to support Jones' (1986) contention that performance differences with a given submaximum resistance may be due to inherent physiological characteristics. It is possible that differences in muscle fiber types may be a factor in the number of repetitions completed with a given submaximum weightload.

Summary

As a result of widely published strength training guidelines, many participants follow an 8–12 repetition training protocol. However, individuals who have low levels of muscle endurance may achieve better results by training with fewer repetitions, and individuals who have high levels of muscle endurance may attain better results by training with more repetitions. It is recommended that most people train with a given weightload until 12 repetitions can be performed, at which time the weightload should be increased by about 5 percent.

EFFECTS OF DIFFERENT TRAINING SPEEDS ON STRENGTH DEVELOPMENT

When assisting muscles are utilized to initiate movements, more weight can be lifted at fast speeds than at slow speeds. Consequently, many people associate fast training with muscle strength. However, because faster lifting movements involve more momentum, it is important to determine whether muscle force actually increases or decreases with faster movement speeds.

Westcott (1984b) observed that when momentum is neutralized by means of isokinetic strength testing equipment, muscles always produce more force at slow movement speeds than fast movement speeds. In numerous Cybex evaluations of athletes, nonathletes, males, females, older persons, and younger persons, the pattern of muscle force production is always the same. Maximum muscle force invariably decreases as the speed of movement increases. As illustrated in Figure 5–5, the subject produced a maximum quadriceps force of 168 pounds at the relatively slow movement speed of 60 degrees per second. When the movement speed was increased to 120 degrees per second his quadriceps force was only 120 pounds. Increasing the movement speed to 180 degrees per second reduced his maximum quadriceps strength to 94 pounds.

This observation indicates that momentum must play a major role in fast lifting movements. In fact, it would appear that there is a direct relationship between movement speed and momentum and an inverse relationship between movement speed and muscle force.

Moffroid and Whipple's Study

In 1970, Moffroid and Whipple compared the effects of two movement speeds on muscle strength. One group of subjects performed an isokinetic knee extension at a speed of 36 degrees per second. Another group of subjects performed an isokinetic knee extension at a speed of 108 degrees per second. Their results showed that the slower trained subjects made greater strength gains when tested at the slower speed, and that the faster trained subjects made greater strength gains when tested at

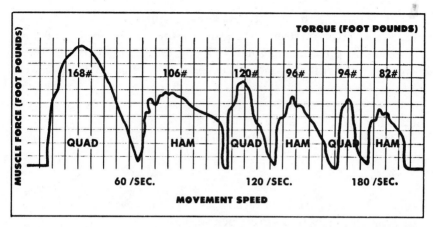

Figure 5–5. Cybex II evaluation of maximum knee extensor and knee flexor strength at speeds of 60, 120, and 180 degrees per second. Note that maximum force production decreases as movement speed increases.

the faster speed. Because these findings revealed a specificity of training effect, it is difficult to draw conclusions regarding the superiority of either training technique for developing muscle strength.

In an attempt to reduce hard to control variables between training groups, Westcott (1986a) conducted a study in which all subjects received both experimental treatments. Each participant trained one leg at a relatively slow speed (60 degrees per second) and the other leg at a relatively fast speed (240 degrees per second).

Six women between 18 and 36 years of age served as subjects in this investigation. All of the women were healthy, physically active individuals who did not engage in any strength training activities before or during the study. Each subject was introduced to the knee extension movement on the computerized Cybex II isokinetic strength testing and training unit. After several practice trials, each leg was tested for maximum strength at 60 degrees per second and 240 degrees per second.

All subjects followed the same strength training protocol. Upon securing the left leg to the training apparatus, they performed 20 seconds of knee extensions at 60 degrees per second. The subjects completed three sets of exercise with a 40-second recovery period between sets. Upon securing the right leg to the training apparatus, they performed 20 seconds of knee extensions at 240 degrees per second. The subjects again completed three sets of exercise with a 40-second recovery period between sets.

After training three times per week for three weeks, each leg was retested for maximum strength at 60 degrees per second and 240 degrees per second. As presented in Table 5−7, only the slow-trained leg showed a strength gain at the slow-movement speed. As presented in Table 5−8, only the slow-trained leg showed a strength gain at the fast movement speed. Dependent t-tests revealed that these strength improvements were statistically significant at the .05 level of probability.

The results of this study indicated that training at 60 degrees per second is more effective than training at 240 degrees per second

Table 5−7   Comparison of Strength Gains for Slow-Trained Leg and Fast-Trained Leg at 60 Degrees per Second

Group	Mean Initial Strength	Mean Final Strength	Mean Strength Increase	Mean Percent Increase
Slow-Trained Leg	108 lbs.	118 lbs.	10 lbs.	9%
Fast-Trained Leg	106 lbs.	105 lbs.	None	None

Table 5−8   Comparison of Strength Gains for Slow-Trained Leg and Fast-Trained Leg at 240 Degrees per Second

Group	Mean Initial Strength	Mean Final Strength	Mean Strength Increase	Mean Percent Increase
Slow-Trained Leg	60 lbs.	65 lbs.	5 lbs.	8%
Fast-Trained Leg	63 lbs.	63 lbs.	None	None

for improving muscle strength. Because the slow-trained leg exhibited strength gains at both the slow speed an the fast speed, and because the fast-trained leg failed to increase strength at either speed, there was no apparent specificity of training effect.

As shown in Tables 5–7 and 5–8, the subjects invariably achieved higher strength scores at 60 degrees per second than at 240 degrees per second. Research by Lesmes et al. (1983) has determined that both fast-twitch and slow-twitch muscle fibers are activated during maximum muscle contractions regardless of the movement speed. Consequently, it is unlikely that the difference in strength scores was due to selective recruitment of fast-twitch or slow-twitch muscle fibers. It is suggested that more muscle force can be produced at slow movement speeds because there is more time to activate more muscle fibers, both slow-twitch and fast-twitch.

Summary

These research findings demonstrate that greater muscle force is produced at slow movement speeds. It also appears that slow training is more effective than fast training for developing muscle strength. Slow strength training is characterized by a longer period of muscle tension and more time for muscle fiber recruitment. Fast strength training enables one to use heavier weightloads, but this is due to assisting muscles and momentum rather than more muscle force. It is therefore recommended that strength training repetitions be performed slowly for best results. The slow movement speed utilized in this study, 60 degrees per second, corresponds to a two-second lifting movement for most strength training exercises (i.e., leg extension, leg curl, triceps extension, biceps curl, and other exercises with about 120 degrees of movement range). In addition to producing better strength gains, slow training is much less likely to cause soft tissue injuries (see Chapter 6).

EFFECTS OF DIFFERENT TRAINING TIMES ON STRENGTH DEVELOPMENT

Most people feel that training time is a matter of personal preference with little bearing on one's strength development. Some people seem to function best in the morning, while others tend to be more productive in the evening. Because most sports practice sessions are held after school, athletes grow accustomed to training in the afternoon. Without exploring the area of biorhythms, it would seem to make sense that once a training schedule has been established, one will probably perform best at his or her regular workout time. However, it is also logical to assume that the cumulative effect of general fatigue may influence physical performance later in the day.

Westcott (1986j) decided to test this hypothesis on an important muscle group that typically works 16 hours a day, even while driving the car, sitting in the office, or studying in the library. The trapezius and posterior neck muscles maintain the head in an erect posture throughout one's working hours. Needless to say, the neck extensors are key muscles with regards to safety and performance in sports such as football and wrestling.

The subjects in this study were six men and four women who were already engaged in a strength training program. All of the participants had sedentary occupations that required a minimum amount of physical exertion. Each subject was evaluated for neck extension strength on a Nautilus neck machine with a weightload that could be lifted at least ten repetitions. The subjects were randomly tested with the same weightload before 10:00 A.M. and after 5:00 P.M. on nonconsecutive days.

The results showed that the subjects completed 44 percent more repetitions in the morning session than in the evening session (see Figure 5−6). The morning performance exceeded the evening performance in every case, even though many of the subjects normally trained later in the day.

These statistically significant findings suggest that daily fatigue may have a profound effect on the neck extensor muscles. It would appear that holding one's head in an upright position for several hours a day may reduce neck strength substantially.

Although other muscle groups may not experience as much strength loss during the course of a day, it is possible that overall muscle performance may be higher during the morning hours for many people. From a practical perspective, business persons who have the option of strength training before work should experiment with a morning workout. Perhaps more importantly, football players, wrestlers, and other athletes may benefit from a before-school strength training program with regards to neck conditioning.

Summary

In accordance with the Principle of Rebuilding Time (Chapter 4), one should take a workout at the peak of the muscle-rebuilding phase to

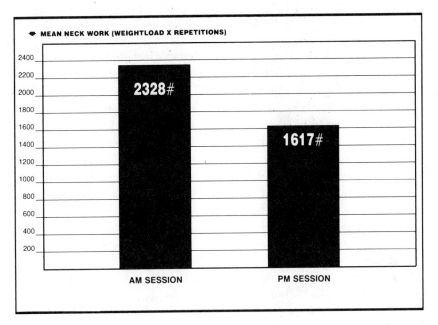

Figure 5-6. Comparison of A.M. Results and P.M. Results with Neck Extensor Exercise.

obtain maximum strength benefits. Similarly, one should train when both the energy level and strength level are highest for best results. These findings indicate that the neck extensor muscles perform significantly better at the beginning of the day than at the end of the day. It is therefore recommended that neck strengthening exercises be performed during the morning hours when the general fatigue level is lower. It is suggested that morning strength workouts may produce excellent overall results for the same reason, but individual training preferences should certainly be taken into consideration.

EFFECTS OF STRENGTH TRAINING ON BLOOD PRESSURE

There is a common misconception that strength training has an adverse affect on blood pressure. Although exercise physiologists are well aware that isometric strength training can cause unusually large increases in systolic and diastolic blood pressures, there is considerably less information on blood pressure response to isotonic strength training (Astrand,

1977; Karpovich and Sinning, 1971; Lamb, 1978; Mathews and Fox, 1976; Pollock, Wilmore, and Fox, 1978).

Recent studies of blood pressure changes during isotonic strength training have produced different results. MacDougall et al. (1983) found extremely high systolic and diastolic blood pressures in body builders during heavy leg exercises. In one of the subjects, the intra-arterial blood pressure measured 400/300 mmHg. It is possible that other factors, such a essential hypertension, use of anabolic steroids, and excessive body mass, may have been at least partly responsible for the unusually high blood pressure response (Hunter and McCarthy, 1982; Wright, 1978).

Freedson, Chang, and Katch (1984) reported blood pressures around 240/155 mmHg during free weight and hydraulic bench press exercises. These readings were lower than MacDougall's (1983) readings, but higher than those obtained by Westcott and Howes (1983) and Westcott (1986b).

Westcott and Howes (1983) studied blood pressure response during one-arm biceps curls with light, medium, and heavy weightloads. Blood pressures were monitored throughout each 10-repetition exercise set by means of a sphygmomanometer and stethoscope on the nonexercising arm. The subjects were 24 men and women who had no medical history of cardiovascular disease.

The mean systolic blood pressure increased gradually from 123 mmHg at rest to 165 mmHg during the final repetition with the 10RM weightload. The mean diastolic pressure measured 75 mmHg both before and immediately after the exercise set. Figure 5–7 shows that the systolic blood pressure response was directly related to the training intensity. The peak systolic readings were 143 mmHg with the light weightload, 151 mmHg with the medium weightload, and 165 mmHg with the heavy weightload.

Sex comparisons revealed higher systolic blood pressures for the male subjects, and age comparisons revealed higher systolic blood pressures for the subjects over 38 years of age (see Table 5–9).

Based on the findings of this study, it would appear that one-arm biceps curls performed with the 10RM weightload do not produce abrupt, excessive, or unusual blood pressure responses. In fact, the 34 percent increase in systolic pressure (see Figure 5–8) compared favorably with a 35 percent increase in systolic pressure measured on 23 subjects during stationary cycling (see Figure 5–9).

Because lower body exercises involve more muscle mass and more muscle force than upper body exercises, Westcott (1986b) examined

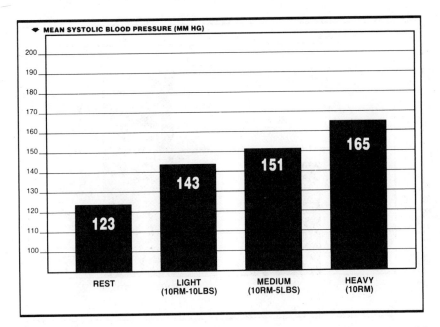

Figure 5-7. Systolic Blood Pressures at Rest and During Final Repetition with Light, Medium, and Heavy Weightloads.

Table 5-9 Mean Systolic Blood Pressure Responses During 10-Repetition Sets of One-Arm Dumbbell Curls (N=24)

Subjects	Resting Systolic Pressure	Peak Systolic Pressure	Percent Increase
All	123	165	34%
Males	131	179	37%
Females	114	148	29%
Over 38	132	175	33%
Under 38	115	154	34%

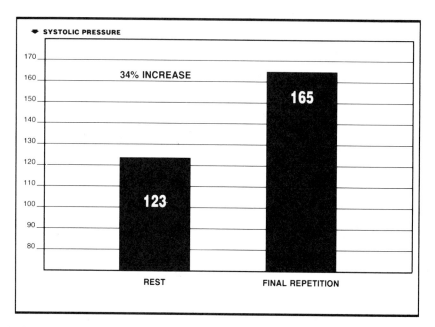

Figure 5–8. Systolic Blood Pressure Response During 10RM Exercise Set One-Arm Curls (N=24).

blood pressure response during Nautilus duo-squats with heavy weight-loads. Blood pressures were monitored throughout each 10-repetition exercise set by means of a sphygmomanometer and stethoscope on the right arm. The subjects were 25 men and women with no medical history of cardiovascular disease.

The mean systolic blood pressure increased gradually from 127 mmHg at rest to 190 mmHg during the final repetition with the 10RM weightload. The mean diastolic pressure measured 73 mmHg before and 61 mmHg immediately after the exercise set.

Sex comparisons revealed higher systolic pressures for the male participants, and age comparisons revealed higher systolic pressures for the subjects over 38 years of age (see Table 5–10).

Although the Nautilus duo-squats produced a 50 percent increase in systolic blood pressure (see Figure 5–10), the response pattern was similar to the one-arm biceps curls. All of the subjects demonstrated a gradual, progressive, and predictable systolic pressure increase during the 10-repetition exercise sets. It is noted that a systolic pressure of 190 mmHg is not uncommon during vigorous physical activity, and few exercises are as demanding as the Nautilus duo-squat.

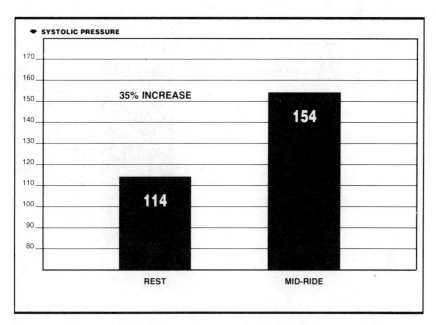

Figure 5-9. Systolic Blood Pressure Response During Stationary Cycling (N=23).

Table 5-10 Mean Systolic Blood Pressure Responses During 10-Repetition Sets of Nautilus Duo-Squats (N=25)

Subjects	Resting Systolic Pressure	Peak Systolic Pressure	Percent Increase
All	127	190	50%
Males	130	195	50%
Females	115	170	48%
Over 38	125	193	54%
Under 38	129	188	46%

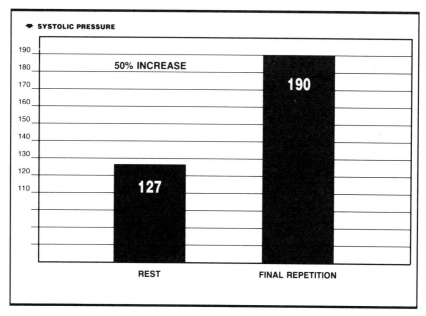

Figure 5-10. Systolic Blood Pressure Response During 10RM Exercise Set Nautilus Duo-Squats (N=25).

Circuit Strength Training

Westcott (1986c) examined the immediate effects of circuit strength training on blood pressure. One hundred men and women participated in this study. The subjects performed one set of 8-12 repetitions on the following Nautilus machines: (1) leg extension, (2) leg curl, (3) hip adduction, (4) hip abduction, (5) low back, (6) abdominal, (7) 10-degree chest, (8) back pullover, (9) lateral raise, (10) biceps, and (11) triceps. The subjects' standing blood pressures were recorded 30-60 seconds before and 30-60 seconds after performing the 11-station exercise circuit.

As presented in Table 5-11, the subjects' mean training time was 29 minutes. Their mean blood pressure 30-60 seconds before the exercise session was 115/67 mmHg, and their mean blood pressure 30-60 seconds after the exercise session was 117/65 mmHg. The 72 male subjects had a mean pre-exercise blood pressure of 118/69 mmHg and a mean post-exercise blood pressure of 119/67 mmHg. The 28 female subjects had a mean pre-exercise blood pressure of 107/62 mmHg and a mean post-exercise blood pressure of 113/59 mmHg.

Table 5-11 Blood Pressure Readings for 72 Men and 28 Women Before and After Completing Nautilus Strength Training Session

	Age (yrs.)	Training Time (Mins.)	Systolic Before (mmHg)	Systolic After (mmHg)	Diastolic Before (mmHg)	Diastolic After (mmHg)
Men	38.3 ± 12.3	28.6 ± 6.7	117.8 ± 10.2	118.5 ± 23.4	69.3 ± 8.8	66.8 ± 14.1*
Women	33.9 ± 11.7	29.4 ± 6.7	107.4 ± 15.2	113.0 ± 10.9*	62.1 ± 10.3	58.9 ± 11.4*
Total	37.0 ± 12.2	28.8 ± 6.7	114.9 ± 12.6	117.0 ± 23.0*	67.3 ± 9.8	64.6 ± 13.8*

*Significantly different from before training session (P<0.05).

The results of this study indicate that the immediate effects of a 29-minute circuit strength training session are a small increase in systolic pressure and a small decrease in diastolic pressure. The increase in systolic pressure and the decrease in diastolic pressure are normal cardiovascular responses to vigorous exercise. It is noted that the participants in this study, most of whom had performed regular circuit strength training for over a year, recorded relatively low blood pressures both before (115/67 mmHg) and after (117/65 mmHg) the exercise session.

Summary

The subjects in Westcott's studies experienced a 35−50 percent increase in systolic blood pressure during a 10-repetition exercise set. After completing an 11-station exercise session, the subjects recorded a small increase in systolic blood pressure and a small decrease in diastolic blood pressure. These results indicate that sensible strength training does not have an adverse affect on blood pressure in healthy adults.

In these studies, sensible strength training was characterized by: (1) weightloads that could be lifted for 10 repetitions, (2) continuous breathing throughout the exercise set, (3) controlled muscle movement throughout the exercise set, and (4) loose handgrips. It must be emphasized that maximum weightloads, breath-holding, static (isometric) contractions, and tight handgrips can produce excessive blood pressure responses.

It is recommended that persons with elevated blood pressures or other cardiovascular abnormalities consult their physician before starting a strength training program. It is also suggested that all participants have periodic blood pressure checks before, during, and after strength training.

EFFECTS OF STRENGTH TRAINING ON HEART RATE

Whenever the demand for energy increases, the heart rate increases. The heart is similar to the fuel pump in an automobile, and the muscles are analogous to the engine. As the muscles perform work, the heart must pump blood to the work site to replenish energy supplies and remove metabolic waste products. Because the heart pumps blood throughout the entire body, activity in any of the major muscle groups will produce a faster heart rate. Although more oxygen is consumed by larger muscle groups, the heart rate response is essentially the same for a leg extension and an arm extension (Hempel and Wells, 1985).

Westcott (1985b) found a gradual and progressive increase in heart rate during 10 repetitions with the 10RM weightload. The mean heart rate response to various exercises for the legs, midsection, torso, and arms rose from about 75 beats per minute at rest to about 130 beats per minute during the final repetition. When subjects took 90-second rests between successive exercises on ten Nautilus machines, the mean heart rate was 128 beats per minute. As the rest intervals between machines decreased to 60 seconds and 30 seconds, the mean heart rates increased to 139 beats per minute and 148 beats per minute, respectively (see Figure 5–11). These results demonstrate that shorter rest periods between exercises produced higher heart rates throughout the training session.

Summary

The heart rate response and systolic blood pressure response to isotonic strength training are similar in that both increase gradually, progressively, and predictably during an exercise set. Ten repetitions

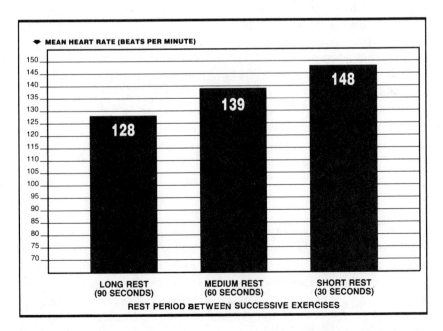

Figure 5–11. Exercise Heart Rates for Ten-Station Workout with Long, Medium, and Short Rests Between Successive Exercises.

with the 10RM weightload typically raise the heart rate from a resting level of 75 beats per minute to a peak level of 130–150 beats per minute. The less rest one takes between exercises, the higher the mean heart rate response. Subjects who rested 30 seconds between ten successive Nautilus exercises experienced a mean heart rate of about 150 beats per minute.

EFFECTS OF STRENGTH TRAINING ON CARDIOVASCULAR PERFORMANCE

Cardiovascular endurance is usually improved when one regularly performs 10–30 minutes of continuous large muscle activity at an intensity sufficient to keep the heart rate above 70 percent of maximum (Zohman, 1974). Darden (1985) has stated that Nautilus strength training meets the criteria for enhancing cardiovascular endurance when the exerciser moves quickly from machine to machine, thereby maintaining a relatively high heart rate throughout the training session.

According to Hurley et al. (1984) and Hempel and Wells (1985), even though Nautilus training can maintain relatively high heart rates, it does not use a high enough percentage of maximum oxygen uptake to produce cardiovascular adaptations. However, Messier and Dill (1985) found a significant increase in maximum oxygen consumption after ten weeks of "short rest" Nautilus training. In fact, the Nautilus participants improved their maximum oxygen consumption as much as the subjects who participated in a running program. Other investigators (Peterson, 1976; Stone et al., 1983; and Goldberg et al., 1983) found significant reductions in the subjects' double product (heart rate × systolic blood pressure) after regular participation in a weight training program. Their findings suggest that the weight training had a positive effect on the subjects' cardiovascular systems.

Westcott and Warren (1985) examined the effects of "short rest" strength training on cardiovascular performance. The subjects, six untrained and sedentary women between 19 and 32 years of age, agreed to perform no physical activity except for the scheduled strength training sessions. They trained three times per week for four weeks. During each training session the subjects completed one set of 8 to 15 repetitions on ten Nautilus machines. The subjects performed their repetitions slowly but moved quickly from machine to machine. The mean training time was 13 minutes, and the mean transition time between machines was about 15 seconds. The subjects were monitored continuously with an electronic heart rate device and reached a mean heart rate of 145 beats per minute at each of the ten exercise stations.

Two days before and two days after the Nautilus training program, the subjects were evaluated for cardiovascular performance on a standard cycle ergometer test. Cardiovascular performance was assessed by the subjects' energy expenditure in METS at 80 percent of maximum heart rate. One MET is equivalent to 3.5 millimeters of oxygen utilization per kilogram of bodyweight per minute.

The subjects' mean pre-training energy output at 80 percent of maximum heart rate was 7.0 METS. After completing 12 "short rest" Nautilus sessions, the subjects' mean energy output at 80 percent of maximum heart rate was 8.3 METS (see Figure 5−12). This represented a 19 percent improvement in cardiovascular performance on the standard cycle ergometer test.

The ability to perform vigorous physical activity is influenced by several interrelated factors, including muscle strength and cardiovascular endurance. The subjects in this study definitely improved their muscle strength, as demonstrated by a 52 percent mean increase in their exercise weightloads.

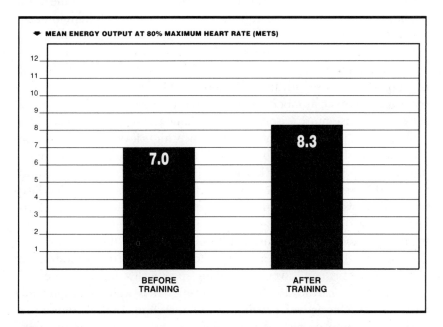

Figure 5−12. Energy Output in METS at 80 Percent of Maximum Heart Rate Before and After "Short Rest" Nautilus Training.

The "short rest" Nautilus program also met the minimum requirements for improving cardiovascular endurance. The subjects performed large muscle activity that maintained their heart rates at 75 percent of maximum for 13 minutes, three days per week for four weeks. It is therefore likely that the participants obtained some cardiovascular benefits, especially since they began the program with relatively low levels of cardiovascular fitness.

Due to the limitations of this study, it cannot be stated that the "short rest" Nautilus training improved the subjects' aerobic capacity. However, the findings do indicate that the "short rest" Nautilus training improved the subjects' capacity to perform aerobic activity.

Although research on the aerobic benefits of strength training is mixed (Hempel and Wells, 1985; Hurley, 1984; Messier and Dill, 1985), other cardiovascular adaptations have been observed. Several investigators have reported increased left ventricle wall thickness as a result of progressive strength training (Ricci et al., 1982; Morganroth et al., 1975; Mathews and Fox, 1976; Fox, 1979). There is also evidence that progressive strength training increases muscle capillarization (McDonagh et al., 1984; Schantz, 1982). These beneficial physiological changes, a stronger pump and a better delivery system, may account for some of the cardiovascular performance improvement associated with high intensity strength training (Peterson, 1976; Westcott and Warren, 1985).

It should be noted that oxygen consumption (Hempel and Wells, 1985) may not be the most appropriate means of assessing cardiovascular function during strength training exercise. Oxygen consumption is directly related to the number of major muscle groups involved in a physical activity. Because muscle isolation is fundamental to successful strength training, one will not normally experience high levels of oxygen consumption during a strength workout. However, whenever any major muscle group performs work, the cardiovascular system responds with increased heart rate, increased blood pressure, and increased blood distribution. It would appear that these responses provide the stimuli for beneficial cardiovascular adaptations, particularly when the heart rate is maintained above 70 percent of maximum for more than 15 minutes.

Finally, the author does not want to imply that strength training in general or "short rest" strength training specifically should be used for the purpose of cardiovascular conditioning. It is well-established that rhythmic, aerobic activities such as jogging, cycling, and swimming produce the greatest cardiovascular benefits (American College of Sports Medicine, 1982). However, there seem to be at least two practical applications for "short rest" strength training. One is during recovery from injuries that prohibit weight-bearing activity. Because all of the major muscle groups can be worked from a supported position (sitting or lying) on Nautilus equipment, "short rest" Nautilus training provides an exercise alternative that includes both muscle strength and cardiovascular endurance components.

The other practical application for "short rest" strength training is the busy individual who has just enough time for three 20-minute exercise sessions per week. The results of Westcott and Warren's (1985) study indicate that "short rest" strength training is an effective means for attaining improvements in both muscle strength and cardiovascular endurance with relatively brief workouts.

Summary

Some research indicates that "short rest" strength training does not improve maximum oxygen consumption, while other research shows a significant improvement in maximum oxygen consumption. Several researchers have observed increased left ventricle mass and increased muscle capillarization in strength trained individuals. The subjects in one study experienced 19 percent improvement in a cardiovascular performance test after four week of "short rest" Nautilus training. These results indicate that "short rest" strength training can improve one's capacity to perform aerobic activity. Although not the preferred method of cardiovascular conditioning, "short rest" strength training that keeps one's heart rate above 70 percent of maximum for 15–20 minutes seems to have some cardiovascular performance benefit.

EFFECTS OF STRENGTH TRAINING ON MUSCLE PERFORMANCE

Most people who begin a strength fitness program are encouraged by the relatively large strength gains they experience during the first few weeks of training. Beginners frequently increase their strength by 40–70 percent after one month of regular workouts (Westcott, 1984a; Westcott and Warren, 1985). Unfortunately, the rate of improvement tends to drop off sharply during the second month of training.

Westcott (1985c) observed six female subjects during eight weeks of supervised strength training. The subjects were evaluated for muscle strength (10RM) at the beginning, midpoint, and end of the training program. All participants performed five exercises, three days per week throughout the course of the study.

As illustrated in Figure 5–13, the women increased their overall muscle strength 76 percent during the first month, and 13 percent during the second month. Although the subjects made 100 percent improvement after eight weeks of training, most of the strength gain occurred during the first month. It has been suggested that much of the initial strength improvement is due to learning factors in the nervous system (McDonagh and Davies, 1984). That is, the early strength gains may be largely due to more efficient use of existing muscle rather than the addition of new muscle.

Westcott (1985d) compared performance improvement on selected weight training machines to strength gains measured on computerized strength testing equipment. The subjects were tested for maximum leg extension strength and maximum leg flexion strength on a Cybex II apparatus. They were also tested for the 10-repetition maximum weight-load (10RM) on a Nautilus Leg Extension Machine and Nautilus Leg Curl

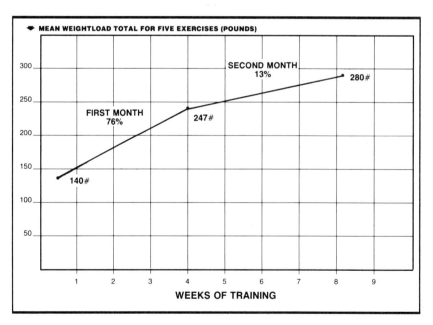

Figure 5–13. Percent Improvement During First and Second Months of Training.

Machine. The subjects trained three days per week for four weeks. The training protocol was one set of 8 to 12 repetitions on each of the Nautilus machines with a 5 percent weight increase whenever 12 repetitions were completed. Two days after the final training session, the subjects were again evaluated for maximum leg extension strength and maximum leg flexion strength on the Cybex II apparatus. The same movement pattern and movement speed (60 degrees per second) were used in all of the testing and training sessions.

As shown in Figure 5−14, the performance improvements observed on the Nautilus machines were much greater than the strength gains determined by the computerized strength tests. The subjects increased their 10 repetition maximum weightloads by about 70 percent but improved their maximum strength measurements by less than 10 percent.

These findings indicate that factors other than strength may have been partly responsible for the relatively large performance increases achieved on the Nautilus machines. Factors such as familiarity with the machines, technique adaptations, and more efficient recruitment of muscle fibers undoubtedly contributed to the improved training perfor-

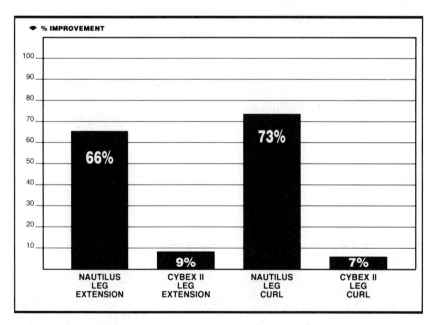

Figure 5−14. Comparison of Strength Improvement on Nautilus Exercises and Cybex II Tests.

mance. It would appear that one learns to use the muscles more effectively when a specific exercise is practiced regularly. Initial performance improvement seems to be influenced more by better utilization of available muscle tissue than by the development of new muscle tissue (Ikai and Fukunaga, 1970; Hakkinen and Komi, 1983; Moritani and DeVries, 1979). Conversely, neurological factors probably play a less significant role in subsequent performance improvement. The smaller gains attained later in the training program, though less prolific, more likely represent new muscle development.

Summary

Most strength training participants experience relatively large increases in their performance levels during the first month of training. Progress usually slows markedly after four weeks, however, and may be a source of discouragement. Research indicates that much of the initial performance improvement is due to neurological factors. Practice enhances neurological efficiency and enables the exerciser to use available muscle tissue more effectively. Subsequent strength gains may come more slowly but are largely due to the development of new muscle tissue.

From a practical standpoint, persons who are aware of the learning factor may be less likely to give up when strength gains come more slowly. They should realize that the smaller improvements experienced later in the training program more accurately represent new muscle strength and should be encouraged by gradual progress.

EFFECTS OF STRENGTH TRAINING ON BODY COMPOSITION

Body composition refers to the ratio of fat weight to lean body weight. Many fitness authorities (Myers, 1975; Golding et al., 1982) recommend that men should have about 15 percent fat weight and women should have about 20 percent fat weight. If asked how to best reduce percent body fat, most people would suggest a low-calorie diet. Unfortunately, research indicates that cutting calories without exercise has some undesirable effects. One result of dieting alone is a decrease in metabolic rate (Clark, 1985). Apparently, the body adapts to fewer food calories by slowing down its rate of energy production. Another result of dieting alone is a loss of lean body weight including muscle tissue, organ tissue, and extracellular fluid (Darden, 1981). It seems that when the caloric supply is diminished, the body draws upon both fat sources and functional tissue for energy requirements.

Most physiologists, nutritionists, and physicians agree that a sensible exercise program should accompany a sound reducing diet for best results. Exercise tends to maintain one's normal metabolic rate and lessen the loss of lean body tissue. In addition, exercise utilizes calories, which facilitates weight reduction. However, the type of exercise one performs has considerable bearing on physiological responses.

Many people believe that aerobic activity is best for losing weight because it burns large amounts of calories. Jogging, bicycling, and swimming may consume an additional 10–15 calories per minute (Astrand, 1977) while one is exercising. However, shortly after the exercise session, one's metabolism returns to normal. A 20-minute run would therefore use about 300 more calories per day than performing no exercise.

Darden (1985) has stated that strength training is a more effective means of losing weight because it burns extra calories while one is exercising and also while one is at rest. He believes the additional muscle that results from strength training increases resting metabolic rate, because muscle tissue has high energy requirements. Lamb (1985) and Johnson (1986) agree that muscle maintenance is a major function of our resting metabolism.

It has therefore been suggested that strength training has a double reducing effect (Darden, 1985). A 20-minute circuit strength training workout burns about 200 calories (Wilmore et al., 1978), which is fewer calories than a 20-minute run burns. However, if as a result of regular strength training one adds two pounds of muscle, additional calories will be used 24 hours a day to meet the increased metabolic requirements.

Westcott (1986d) compared body composition changes for 72 male and female participants in a weight-loss research program. All of the subjects were advised to lose one pound per week through a combination of a low-fat diet and regular exercise. The diet program was based on 20 percent fat intake, 20 percent protein intake, and 60 percent carbohydrate intake. The exercise program was based on three 30-minute training sessions per week for a period of eight weeks.

Twenty-two subjects performed 30 minutes of endurance training (cycling, jogging, or aerobic dance) during each exercise session, and 50 subjects performed 15 minutes of strength training and 15 minutes of endurance training during each exercise session.

At the completion of the program, the subjects who did not do strength training recorded a mean fat loss of 3.0 pounds and a mean muscle loss of 0.5 pounds, for a mean weight loss of 3.5 pounds. The subjects who did perform strength training experienced a mean fat loss of 10.0 pounds and a mean muscle gain of 2.0 pounds for a mean weight loss of 8.0 pounds. The latter results represented a 12-pound improvement in physical appearance (see Table 5–12).

Summary

These findings indicate that strength training is compatible with weight loss. In fact, the subjects who performed strength training experienced greater weight loss and greater fat loss than the subjects who did only aerobic exercise. Because the strength trained subjects simultaneously lost fat weight and gained muscle weight, it would appear that strength training is a highly effective means for improving body composition and physical appearance.

SUMMARY OF RESEARCH ON STRENGTH TRAINING

The research results presented in this chapter are summarized in the following paragraphs. In addition, a statement on implementing the research findings is included to assist in program design and development.

1. *Effects of different training frequencies on strength development.* The research indicates that frequent, short-duration training sessions are more effective than infrequent, long-duration training sessions. It is suggested that excellent results are obtained by both three-day-a-week and two-day-a-week strength training programs.

2. *Effects of different training sets on strength development.* The essential stimulus for strength improvement appears to be a single exercise set performed with near maximum resistance. One study revealed no differences between one-set training and two-set training with regards to strength development. It is suggested that one hard set of exercise for each major muscle group is the most efficient means of strength training.

3. *Effects of different training repetitions on strength development.* Research indicates that most participants obtain excellent strength results by training with 8–12 repetitions per exercise. However, it is possible that

Table 5—12 Mean Changes in Bodyweight, Fat, and Muscle for Weight Loss Participants Who Did Strength Training and Weight Loss Participants Who Did Endurance Training

Subjects	Bodyweight	Fat	Muscle
Strength Trained (n=50)	−8.0	−10.0	+2.0
Endurance (Trained (n=22)	−3.5	−3.0	−0.5

people with low muscle endurance may make better progress by training with fewer repetitions, and people with high muscle endurance may make better progress by training with more repetitions. In general, it is recommended that one train with a weightload that can be performed about 10 times. When 12 repetitions can be completed, the weight load should be increased by about 5 percent.

4. *Effects of different training speeds on strength development.* Greater muscle force is produced at slow movement speeds than at fast movement speeds. Westcott's research revealed that slow strength training is more effective than fast strength training for improving muscle strength. Movement speeds of about 60 degrees per second are recommended for most strength training exercises. This corresponds to approximately two seconds for each lifting movement.

5. *Effects of different training times on strength development.* For best results, one should train when both the energy level and strength level are highest. One researcher discovered that neck extensor strength was significantly higher in the morning than in the evening. Although other muscle groups may be less affected by general fatigue, it is suggested that persons consider training early in the day if at all feasible.

6. *Effects of strength training on blood pressure.* Although studies on blood pressure response to strength training are somewhat conflicting, standard isotonic strength training does not seem to cause unusual or excessive blood pressures. Researchers found a 34 percent increase in systolic blood pressure during an arm exercise and a 50 percent increase in systolic blood pressure during a leg exercise. These blood pressure readings are similar to those recorded during aerobic activities such as jogging and cycling. One investigator recorded a small increase in systolic blood pressure and a small decrease in diastolic blood pressure immediately after a 29-minute circuit strength training program. These findings indicate that sensible strength training does not produce adverse blood pressure responses and is a relatively safe activity for healthy individuals.

7. *Effects of strength training on heart rate.* Like systolic blood pressure, heart rate increases gradually, progressively, and predictably during an exercise set. Persons who take very brief rests between successive exercise stations may maintain heart rates at around 150 beats per minute throughout the training session.

8. *Effects of strength training on cardiovascular performance.* The subjects in one study demonstrated a 19 percent improvement on a cardiovascular performance test after four weeks of "short rest" strength training. This result indicates that "short rest" strength training may increase one's capacity to perform aerobic activity. Other studies have shown increases in maximum oxygen consumption, left ventricle mass, and muscle capillarization as a result of "short rest" strength training. It is therefore concluded that some cardiovascular performance factors may be improved by strength training in a manner that keeps the heart rate above 70 percent of maximum for 15–20 minutes.

9. *Effects of strength training on muscle performance.* The large performance improvements that occur during the early stages of training are probably due to neurological factors that enable the participant to use available muscle tissue more effectively. The smaller strength gains obtained later in the program are predominantly the result of new muscle tissue. Therefore, one should not be discouraged when progress appears to slow down.

10. *Effects of strength training on body composition.* Weight-loss programs based on dieting and aerobic exercise may result in muscle loss as well as fat loss. Weight-loss programs that include strength training simultaneously increase muscle weight and decrease fat weight, which produces greater improvement in body composition. A low-fat diet reduces caloric intake, and aerobic activity increases caloric expenditure during exercise. However, strength training increases caloric expenditure both during exercise and during rest, because additional muscle tissue requires additional energy supplies for maintenance and repair. Consequently, strength training is an excellent means for improving body composition.

Chapter Six

Designing the Strength Training Program

There are essentially eight factors that should be considered when designing a strength training program. These are: (1) exercise selection, (2) exercise frequency, (3) exercise duration, (4) exercise intensity, (5) exercise speed, (6) exercise range, (7) exercise progression, and (8) exercise continuity. This section will discuss each of these factors in light of the research findings presented in Chapter 5.

EXERCISE SELECTION

One of the biggest problems encountered by strength training enthusiasts is musculoskeletal injuries. One of the most common causes of musculoskeletal injuries is exercise specialization. Many people have misunderstood the principle of training specificity and encountered various overuse injuries as a result.

As discussed in Chapter 4, training specificity implies conditioning the appropriate muscle groups and energy systems for a particular activity. For example, if one wishes to succeed as a sprinter, it would make sense to strengthen the legs and the anaerobic energy system (i.e., the system that provides large amounts of energy for short periods of time). Unfortunately, many track coaches, including the author, have taken this concept one step too far. Because the quadriceps are the dominant muscle group in sprinting, we have often emphasized strength exercises for these muscles and de-emphasized strength exercises for the opposing hamstrings. As a result, the anterior thigh muscles become disproportionately stronger than the posterior thigh muscles. At some point, usually driving off the starting blocks, this muscle imbalance produces a muscle pull as the stronger quadriceps overpower the weaker hamstrings.

The same pattern of injury occurs in the upper body when throwing coaches train the arm extensor muscles harder than the arm flexor muscles. At some point, the force-producing capacity of the overtrained triceps muscles exceeds the force-restraining capacity of the under-trained biceps muscles and results in soft tissue injury.

Finally, how many weight trainers have worked one or two exercises, such as bench presses and curls, to the exclusion of a well-rounded training program? It is easy to recognize those who have trained in this specialized manner by their uneven physical development and their chronic injuries to the shoulder and elbow joints.

The simple solution to each of these problems is to pair the Principle of Training Specificity with the Principle of Muscle Balance (see Chapter 4). In other words, always maintain balanced strength around a joint by training both the prime mover muscle groups and the antagonist muscle groups.

Comprehensive Training

In the opinion of the author, the best way to maximize physical performance and minimize injury potential is to train in a comprehensive manner. That is, perform one exercise for each of the major muscle groups to ensure balanced muscle development.

There are basically 13 major muscle groups and 6 minor muscle groups that should be considered in a comprehensive training program. As illustrated in Figures 6−1 and 6−2, these are as follows:

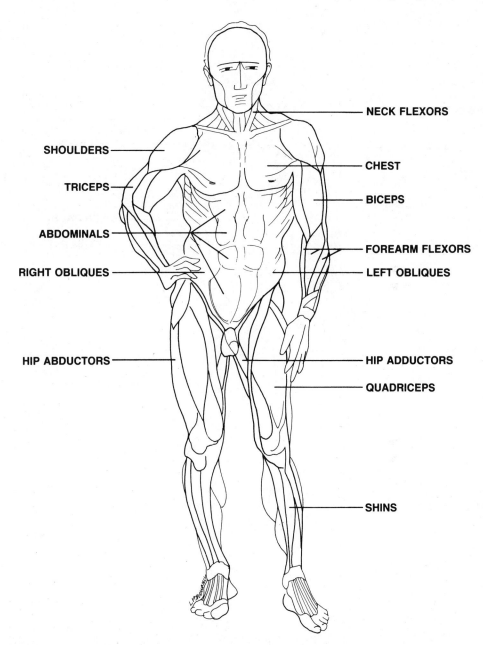

Figure 6-1. Muscles of the Body: Front

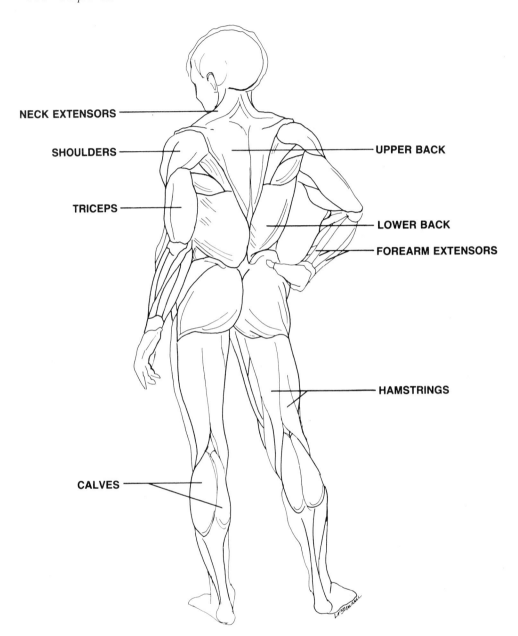

NECK EXTENSORS

SHOULDERS

TRICEPS

UPPER BACK

LOWER BACK

FOREARM EXTENSORS

HAMSTRINGS

CALVES

Figure 6–2.   Muscles of the Body: Back

Major Muscle Groups	*Minor Muscle Groups*
1. Quadriceps	1. Calves
2. Hamstrings	2. Shins
3. Hip Adductors	3. Left Obliques
4. Hip Abductors	4. Right Obliques
5. Lower Back	5. Forearm Flexors
6. Abdominals	6. Forearm Extensors
7. Chest	
8. Upper Back	
9. Shoulders	
10. Biceps	
11. Triceps	
12. Neck Flexors	
13. Neck Extensors	

It is recommended that each of the major muscle groups be trained at least twice per week and that each of the minor muscle groups be worked at least once per week. Many free-weight exercises involve several muscle groups at a time. For example, bar dips, bench presses, and incline presses all utilize the chest muscles, anterior shoulder muscles, triceps muscles, and forearm muscles. Pull-ups, pull-downs, and seated rows all use the upper back muscles, posterior shoulder muscles, biceps muscles, and forearm muscles. On the other hand, persons who train on Nautilus equipment typically work one major muscle group per exercise and must therefore use about 13 machines for a comprehensive conditioning session.

EXERCISE FREQUENCY

Overtraining is an occupational hazard among athletes. Distance runners used to train every other day, then every day, then twice a day. The result has been small decreases in running times and large increases in running injuries. The body needs time to recover from the training stress and to respond to the training stimulus. This is especially true for physical activities that are high intensity in nature. That is, activities that require high levels of force production and high levels of energy production. Strength training and long sprints (440 yards, 880 yards) fall into this category.

Research (Westcott, 1974) indicates that harder workouts require longer recovery periods for the rebuilding processes to occur. Although individual differences must be taken into consideration, most people respond well to a three-day-per-week strength training program unless their workouts are long and laborious. Persons who perform one high-intensity exercise set for each major muscle group typically recover within 48 hours. As illustrated in Figure 6–3, this often represents the height of the rebuilding/overcompensation process and marks the best time for a new training stimulus.

Some people can make continued progress with more frequent strength training sessions, while other people require three days to recuperate from intense workouts. The only way to determine one's ideal recovery time is through trial-and-error experimentation. If the training weightloads feel a little lighter than last time, then the rest period is appropriate. Ideally, one should see some improvement in each successive workout, at least until relatively high strength levels are attained.

Training consistency is essential for optimum strength results. The person who frequently misses workouts will fail to build on the previous

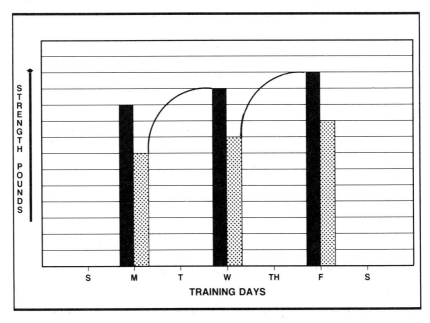

Figure 6–3. Pattern of strength development when recovery period is properly matched to training intensity. When appropriate rest is obtained between training sessions, the muscle rebuilds to a higher strength level.

strength foundation and will allow the deconditioning process to begin prior to the next training session (see Chapter 4). On the other hand, when one takes workouts back to back, the muscles don't have time to regain their previous strength level, let alone become stronger (Westcott, 1985e).

As a training recommendation, beginners are advised to try a three-day-per-week workout program. It is suggested that one train all of the major muscle groups each training day and rest all of the major muscle groups each nontraining day.

EXERCISE DURATION

Exercise duration has two components. The first involves the length of each training set and the second involves the length of each training session. Let's begin with the optimum duration for each training set. As discussed in Chapter 5, training weightloads below 65 percent of maximum may provide little stimulus for strength development. Most people can perform about 15 repetitions with 65 percent of their maximum weightload. Consequently, if one is interested in gaining muscle strength, it is generally not advisable to perform more than 15 repetitions per set of exercise. Assuming that each repetition is executed in 7 seconds, it would take about 105 seconds to complete 15 repetitions. Ninety to 120 seconds is approximately the upper end of the anaerobic energy system. Any physical activity lasting much beyond 90–120 seconds places greater demands on the aerobic energy system.

As an example, sprinters (100 yards, 220 yards, 440 yards, and 880 yards) have a different physical appearance than distance runners (mile, two-mile, six-mile, and marathon). Sprinters typically have highly trained anaerobic energy systems and muscular physiques. On the other hand, distance runners usually have highly trained aerobic energy systems and slender physiques.

Although genetic endowment has a lot to do with one's response to exercise, activity bouts that last more than 90–120 seconds provide less stimulus for strength development. It is therefore recommended that the duration of an exercise set generally not exceed 15 repetitions or 105 seconds.

The heaviest weightload that can be lifted one time provides both maximum muscle stress and maximum risk of injury. Although the 1RM weightload has long been used to demonstrate strength, the high rate of injuries encountered in this type of strength testing makes it a questionable practice at best. Weight lifters use maximum weightloads in competition, but many professional athletic teams evaluate strength by less dangerous methods.

The 10 repetition maximum weightload is often used for strength assessments, and normative data are available through the YMCA (Westcott, Benkis, and McPhee, 1985). Because the 10RM weightload corresponds to about 75 percent of the 1RM weightload for most people, it is a relatively valid and reliable predictor of muscle strength. More importantly, there is much less risk of injury when using the 10RM weightload. First, the lighter resistance places less momentary stress on muscles, tendons, ligaments, and connective tissue. Second, by the time maximum effort is necessary, the muscles have had 50–60 seconds of specific warm-up and are prepared for the final 2 or 3 repetitions.

Training with 5 repetitions represents a compromise between the 1RM and 10RM weightload. There is an intermediate resistance and an intermediate risk of injury. However, 35 seconds of continuous muscle tension (5 repetitions at 7 seconds each) may not be sufficient to stimulate maximum muscle fitness in many participants. It is suggested that one not train with fewer than 5 repetitions, which generally corresponds to about 85 percent of maximum weightload.

Most exercisers can perform about 8 repetitions with 80 percent of their maximum weightload and about 12 repetitions with 70 percent of their maximum weightload. Training within an 8–12 repetition range provides an excellent strength stimulus for most people. At 7 seconds per repetition, this represents about 55–85 seconds of continuous muscle effort. The general repetitions-weightloads relationships are presented in Table 6–1.

Workout Duration

In terms of the workout duration, each training session should be completed as efficiently as possible. In other words, one should take only as much time as necessary to move from exercise to exercise. As discussed in Chapter 5, "short rest" strength training provides important fitness benefits.

If one performs one exercise for each of the 13 major muscle groups, and if each exercise set takes about one minute, then the training session will include 13 minutes of high-intensity activity. If approximately 30 seconds are taken between exercises to record information, adjust

Table 6-1   Relationship Between Various Weightloads, Repetitions, and Training Duration

Percent of Maximum Weightload	Approximate Number of Repetitions	Approximate Training Duration at 7 Seconds per Repetition
85%	5 reps.	35 secs.
80%	8 reps.	55 secs.
75%	10 reps.	70 secs.
70%	12 reps.	85 secs.
65%	15 reps.	105 secs.

weights, etc., then the training session will include 6 minutes of low-intensity activity. The total training time will be just under 20 minutes. If 60-second transition times are required, the workout duration will increase to 25 minutes. It is suggested that a properly conducted strength training session be completed within 20-25 minutes for best overall results.

EXERCISE INTENSITY

Perhaps the single most important factor for strength development is the exercise intensity. The intensity of the work bout provides the essential stimulus for muscle rebuilding and strength improvement. Although intensity is sometimes associated with explosive movements and grimaced faces, this is not the case. Both explosive movements, which utilize momentum, and grimaced faces, which use valuable energy, actually reduce the training intensity.

High-intensity training means pushing one's muscles to the point where they can no longer contract concentrically. In other words, until they are completely fatigued and can no longer move the resistance. This state is sometimes referred to as momentary muscle failure, because the muscles have reached their temporary functional limit.

One can conceivably reach momentary muscle failure by performing one repetition with 300 pounds or by doing 300 repetitions with 10 pounds. However, the former method carries a high risk of injury, and the latter method provides little stimulus for strength gain. As discussed in the last section, 8 to 12 repetitions is a safe and effective training range for most people, as long as the resistance is sufficient to cause momentary muscle failure. This normally requires training with 70−80 percent of maximum weightload.

As an illustration of high-intensity training, assume that during John's last workout he completed 10 repetitions with 75 pounds in the leg extension exercise. Today he also places 75 pounds on the weightstack and begins to exercise. He performs the first 6 repetitions slowly and with moderate effort. Although the 7th and 8th repetitions are difficult, John maintains good form and full movement range. The 9th and 10th repetitions produce considerable discomfort in the quadriceps muscles, and John can no longer attain complete leg extension. He attempts another repetition, but experiences momentary muscle failure and cannot move the weight beyond the midpoint. John does not use other muscle groups, momentum, or poor form to "kick out" the final repetition. He simply squeezes the muscles in a deliberate manner until they are overcome by the resistance. If John had stopped at the completion of 10 repetitions, he would have missed the greatest stimulus for muscle development. By continuing to exercise in good form to the limit of his contractile capacity. John achieved a high-intensity training effect.

Although this type of training is very demanding, it is occasionally desirable to work the muscles even more intensely. One method for making the exercise set even more stressful is to reduce the weightload at the point of momentary muscle failure and force out a few more repetitions with a lighter resistance. This is referred to as breakdown training.

For example, let's assume that John has 100 available muscle fibers, and that each muscle fiber exerts one pound of force. In order to lift 75 pounds in the leg extension, John requires 75 contracting muscle fibers. As John continues to exercise, some muscle fibers fatigue and can no longer exert force. After 10 repetitions perhaps 30 muscle fibers are fatigued, and John can no longer lift the 75 pound weightload. If he immediately reduces the resistance by 20 pounds, he may complete three more repetitions and fatigue another 15 muscle fibers. By so doing, he has hypothetically exhausted 45 of the 100 muscle fibers at the completion of the exercise set.

This is a painful means of training, but it provides a more intense stimulus than performing three sets of 10 repetitions with the same weightload. Resting between sets permits the fatigued fibers to recover. Because each set is discontinued when 75 pounds can no longer be lifted, only about 30 of the 100 muscle fibers ever reach exhaustion even though several sets are performed.

For most purposes, one set of exercise that produces momentary muscle failure between 8 and 12 repetitions is sufficient training stimulus for strength development. However, when greater muscle stimulus is desired, breakdown training offers a controlled means of reaching deeper into one's strength reserves.

Training intensity is only partly related to weightload. If John were to train explosively, he might use 100 pounds instead of 75 pounds in the leg extension. However, momentum, not muscle, would be responsible for lifting the additional 25 pounds. Training with heavier weightloads than one can lift slowly increases the role of momentum and the risk of injury. On the other hand, to minimize the role of momentum and the risk of injury one should train with the lightest weightload that completely exhausts the muscles within 8 to 12 repetitions. That means training slowly and strictly, with full emphasis on the target muscle group rather than assisting muscle groups.

Exercise intensity is the key to efficient strength training. In terms of muscle development, one hard set of exercise is more productive than several sets at submaximum effort. It is therefore recommended that one typically train with a weightload that produces momentary muscle failure within 8 to 12 carefully performed repetitions.

EXERCISE SPEED

The speed at which one performs an exercise may be the second most important factor for safe and effective strength training. There are six reasons that make slow training technique preferable to fast training technique.

More Muscle Tension

First, slow strength training produces a longer period of continuous muscle tension. A slow lifting movement provides a longer period of muscle tension during the concentric contraction, and a slow lowering movement provides a longer period of muscle tension during the eccentric contraction.

For example, a fast-paced, one-second-up and one-second-down training cadence requires only 20 seconds of continuous muscle tension to complete 10 repetitions. On the other hand, a slow-paced, two-second-up and four-second-down training cadence requires 60 seconds of continuous muscle tension to complete 10 repetitions.

Given the same weightload, both methods accomplish the same amount of work. However, the slower technique uses more muscle effort, while the fast technique uses more momentum. Muscle effort is the key to muscle development.

More Muscle Force

Isokinetic evaluations of maximum muscle strength invariably reveal that more muscle force is produced at slower movement speeds. As illustrated in Figure 6−4, there is an inverse relationship between movement speed and muscle force. The maximum muscle force produced at 60 degrees per second is greater than the maximum muscle force produced at 120 degrees per second. Likewise, the maximum muscle force produced at 120 degrees per second is greater than the maximum muscle force produced at 180 degrees per second. Because muscle force decreases as movement speed increases, fast strength training seems counterproductive for maximum strength development (Clarke and Manning, 1985).

More Muscle Fibers

The two basic factors in muscle force production are the number of muscle fibers activated and the firing rate of the motor nerve impulses. Muscle force can be increased by activating more muscle fibers, speeding up the firing rate, or both. Because the firing rate at slow speeds does not exceed the firing rate at fast speeds, the greater muscle force produced at slow speeds is apparently due to greater recruitment of muscle fibers. Research indicates that maximum contractions utilize both fast-twitch and slow-twitch muscle fibers (Lesmes et al., 1983). It therefore appears that slow training provides more time to activate both muscle fiber types, which results in greater force production.

More Muscle Power

Power is the product of force times speed. Power can therefore be enhanced by increasing the muscle force, the movement speed, or both. Both maximum muscle force and maxmium movement speed are neces-

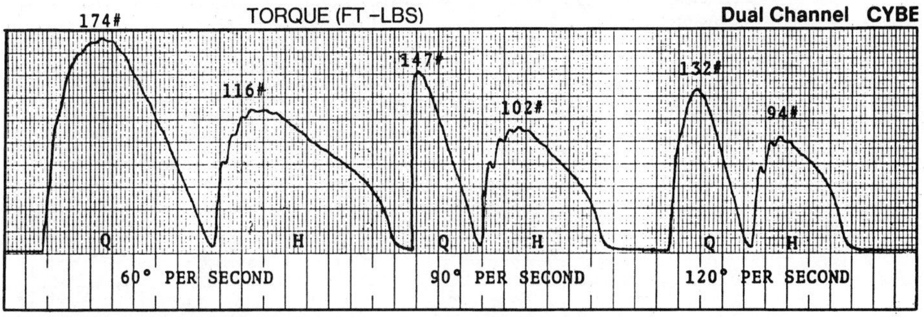

Figure 6–4. Isokinetic Assessment of Muscle Force Production at Various Movement Speeds

sary for maximum power production. However, each component must be trained separately for best results. Combining strength training with speed training is not an effective method for improving either the strength factor or the speed factor.

For example, Susan can perform 10 incline presses with 70 pounds. Her shotput coach recommends that she train with 35 pounds at a much faster cadence to develop her explosiveness. Unfortunately, this type of training will hurt Susan's shotput performance more than it will help. The 35-pound weightload is too light to stimulate strength gains and will probably result in a strength decrement. The 35-pound weightload is four times heavier than the shot and cannot be moved nearly as quickly nor in the same pattern. Consequently, the fast weight training repetitions have no beneficial effect on her movement speed. The most likely outcome from this type of training is soft tissue injury resulting from throwing and catching a 35-pound object.

As shown in Figure 6–5, one can lift heavy weightloads slowly or light weightloads quickly, but one cannot lift heavy weightloads quickly. Because near-maximum resistance is essential for maximum strength development, it is recommended that one train with relatively heavy weightloads and relatively slow speeds to enhance the force factor. As more muscle strength is developed, the force factor increases and permits greater power production.

Less Tissue Trauma

Speed is an essential ingredient in any power event. However, almost all power events are performed with bodyweight (e.g., long jump,

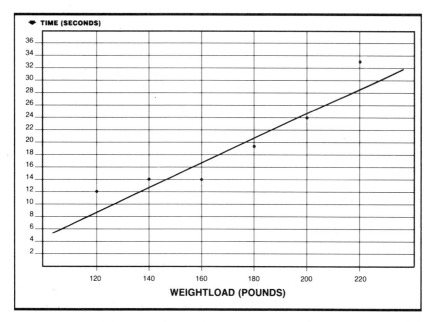

Figure 6-5. Subjects' speed-intensity curve for executing 10 repetitions with various weightloads in the bench press exercise. Note that as the weightload increases, the repetitions are performed more slowly.

high jump) or with relatively light implements (e.g., shot, discus). Power events performed with heavy resistance (e.g., clean and jerk) place great stress on joint structures, thereby increasing the risk of tissue trauma.

The faster one accelerates an object, the greater the initial stress on the involved tendons, ligaments, and muscle fascia. For example, consider attaching a rope from a tow truck to a disabled car. The faster the tow truck accelerates, the greater the stress on the connecting rope and the greater the probability of breaking the rope. Similarly, the faster one decelerates an object, the greater the terminal stress on the involved tendons, ligaments, and muscle fascia. For example, the faster the speed of the tow truck, the greater the difficulty of controlling the disabled car upon stopping quickly.

Slow lifting movements accomplish the same amount of work and produce greater muscle tension than fast lifting movements. However, slow strength training causes less tissue trauma at the start and finish of the exercise movement and is therefore less likely to result in training injuries. For this reason alone, slow strength training should be the preferred technique for physical conditioning programs.

Less Momentum

Momentum plays a part in virtually all weight-training exercises. The faster the lifting movement, the greater the momentum. This is an important consideration because as the momentum component increases, the muscle component decreases. By developing momentum, one can lift heavier weightloads with less sustained muscle effort.

There are many means of generating momentum. The most common technique involves the use of assisting muscle groups to begin the lifting movement (i.e., using the trunk extensor muscles to initiate barbell curls). Although heavier weightloads can be utilized, the target muscle group (biceps) actually receives less training stimulus due to the momentum factor.

Another example of momentum-assisted weight training is bouncing the barbell off the chest during the bench press exercise. In addition to the high injury potential, this careless use of momentum reduces the training effect on the target muscle groups (chest, shoulders, triceps).

While momentum certainly has its place in sporting events, it should play a minor role in strength training programs. Momentum-assisted weight training gives the appearance of greater muscle strength but actually decreases demands on the target muscle groups and increases stress on the joint structures.

Based on these six arguments for slow strength training technique and on the research results presented in Chapter 5, it is recommended that lifting movements not exceed 60 degrees per second. This corresponds to about two seconds for most strength training movements. An exercise with 180 degrees of movement range, such as a Nautilus pullover, should require about three seconds to complete the lifting movement.

Because lowering movements are easier than lifting movements, it is suggested that the lowering phase be performed more slowly than the lifting phase. As a rule of thumb, four seconds provides a safe and effective eccentric contraction. Therefore, six seconds per repetition (two-second lifting movement and four-second lowering movement) is the recommended strength training speed. As will be discussed in the next section, a momentary pause in the fully contracted position may also be advantageous.

EXERCISE RANGE

Almost everyone agrees that it is important to exercise through a full range of movement. The emphasis is usually on stretching the muscle to its full extension in order to prevent loss of flexibility. It is indeed important to fully extend the muscle during the eccentric contraction. However, it is equally important to fully contract the muscle during the concentric contraction. In fact, whenever a particular muscle group is fully contracted, the opposite muscle group is fully stretched.

For example, as one performs a triceps exercise, the triceps muscles shorten and biceps muscles lengthen. At the end point of the exercise, the triceps muscles are in a completely contracted position and the biceps muscles are in a fully stretched position. Conversely, as one performs a biceps exercise, the biceps muscles shorten and the triceps muscles lengthen. At the end point of the exercise, the biceps muscles are in a completely contracted position and the triceps muscles are in a fully stretched position.

Another advantage of performing each repetition to the point of complete muscle contraction is the enhanced stimulus for strength development. A momentary pause in the fully shortened position provides a brief static contraction at the point of near-maximum contact between the actin proteins and the myosin proteins. Due to the mechanics of muscle contraction, this may provide a highly effective stimulus for strength development.

One aspect of exercise range is to select exercises that contract the muscles over a relatively long distance. For example, both the bent row and the pulldown are used to train the latissimus muscles of the upper back. As illustrated in Figures 6–6 through 6–9, the bent row has a movement range of about 90 degrees, and the pulldown has a movement range of about 180 degrees. Because pulldowns stress the latissimus muscles over a longer distance, they are preferable to bent rows, other things being equal.

An equally important aspect of exercise range is to continue each repetition to complete muscle contraction. For example, if John uses 100 pounds, he can achieve full knee extension for 10 repetitions in the leg extension exercise. If John uses 120 pounds, he can achieve full knee extension for only 2 repetitions in the leg extension exercise. The remaining 8 repetitions stop short of full knee extension and do not fully contract the quadriceps muscles. It is more beneficial for Jim to train with full muscle contraction at 100 pounds than with abbreviated muscle contraction at 120 pounds.

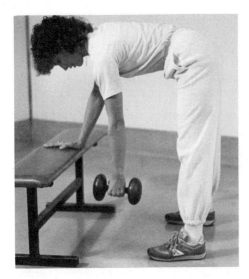

Figure 6–6. Bent Row Start

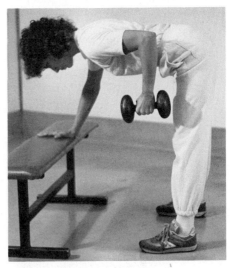

Figure 6–7. Bent Row Finish

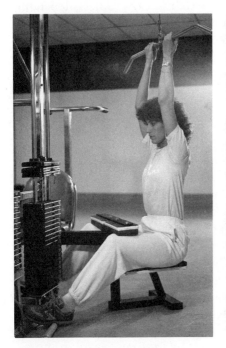

Figure 6–8. Pulldown Start

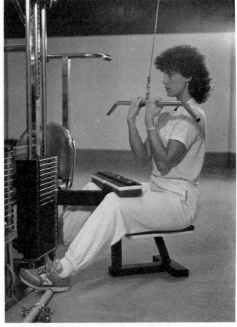

Figure 6–9. Pulldown Finish

Another aspect of exercise range is to begin each repetition from a fully stretched position. For example, many people do not return to a true hang between successive pull-ups. This not only prevents full muscle stretching, but also limits strength development at this end of the movement range.

It is recommended that whenever possible, exercises be performed slowly and smoothly through a complete range of movement. One should not force the muscles into painful positions but should attempt to attain both a fully stretched position and a fully contracted position on each repetition.

EXERCISE PROGRESSION

According to the Stress Adaptation Principle (see Chapter 4), muscles require progressive increases in resistance to stimulate new growth and development. Although the means by which muscles achieve higher strength levels is not well understood, it is clear that too much stress can short-circuit the process and cause tissue injury. In fact, the immediate effect of strength training is some degree of muscle weakness, depending on the imposed training stress. Under proper training conditions, the muscles will be weaker but uninjured after the workout. From this post-training low point, the muscles repair and rebuild to slightly greater strength levels during the following 48 hours.

The purpose of progressive resistance exercise is to maximize strength improvement and to minimize muscle injury. This purpose is best served by a long-range approach to strength development. When one is willing to progress gradually towards a strength goal, the results are generally positive and the setbacks are few. When one is in a hurry to attain strength objectives (e.g., get in top shape before football season, bench press 300 pounds before summer break, etc.), the results may still be positive but the setbacks are more numerous. Figure 6–10 depicts typical progress curves for patient individuals and overanxious individuals. Because most setbacks are in the form of injuries, the eventual result of improper strength training can be chronic impairment.

As indicated in Chapter 5, strength performance improves more slowly after the first few weeks of training. It is therefore not advisable to increase training resistance at regular intervals, such as every two weeks.

Rather, it is recommended that one increase the weightload when it is no longer sufficient to fatigue the muscles within 90 seconds. Because it

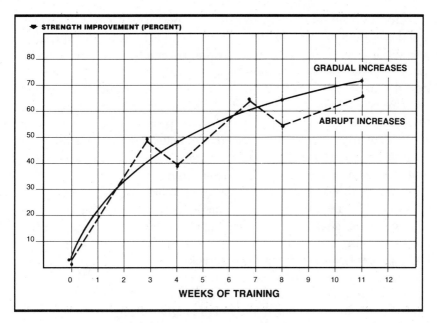

Figure 6-10. Typical Progress Curves for Individuals Who Increase Training Stress Gradually and Individuals Who Increase Training Stress Abruptly

is generally more convenient to count repetitions, it is suggested that one remain at a given resistance until 12 repetitions can be completed in good form. When this is achieved, the weightload should be increased by about 5 percent. One should remain at the new resistance until 12 repetitions can again be performed. This process is referred to as a double progressive training program because one first adds repetitions and then adds resistance. It is a relatively conservative procedure for increasing the training stimulus, but it enables the exerciser to improve consistently with fewer setbacks.

Although the 5 percent incrementation is somewhat arbitrary, it seems to work well based on experience and empirical observation. For example, when George completes 12 repetitions with 100 pounds, he should increase the weightload to 105 pounds the next workout. When Gayle performs 12 repetitions with 50 pounds she should add 2½ pounds the next training session. A 5 percent weightload increase normally results in 2 or 3 fewer repetitions. However, if less than 8 repetitions can be completed, the additional resistance is probably too heavy and should be reduced.

Ideally, one should improve strength performance every workout, and this is often the case during the first few weeks of training. As higher strength levels are attained, however, improvement comes more slowly, and day-to-day fluctuations become more apparent. It is therefore suggested that seasoned strength trainers not expect noticeable strength gains every workout. In fact, strength plateaus are a common occurrence that should be dealt with in a patient and positive manner (Westcott, 1985a). Fortunately, not all muscle groups plateau at the same time, and one can normally see progress in some muscle groups while working on new ways to stimulate stubborn muscle groups.

Five methods for overcoming a strength plateau are: (1) selecting a different exercise for the target muscle group, (2) taking more rest between training sessions, (3) using a lighter resistance and more repetitions, (4) using a heavier resistance and fewer repetitions, and (5) performing breakdown training once a week.

The main point of exercise progression is safety. One must be careful not to progress more rapidly than the muscles' ability to recover from the training stress and to rebuild to a higher strength level. As a rule of thumb, one's total training weightload should increase a little every month even though individual muscle groups may plateau for varying periods of time.

EXERCISE CONTINUITY

Exercise continuity implies an uninterrupted period of large muscle activity such as jogging, swimming, or cycling. Activities such as these maintain an elevated heart rate throughout the training period and promote cardiovascular fitness. On the other hand, activities that require brief bouts of exertion followed by relatively long recovery periods do not maintain elevated heart rates. As usually practiced, weight training is a discontinuous activity involving 30-second work bouts followed by three minute recovery periods. Because the rest periods are relatively long, this type of strength training does not promote much in the way of cardiovascular fitness.

It is possible, however, to conduct strength training in a more continuous manner. For example, let's assume that John performs one set of 10 repetitions for each major muscle group. That is, he works about 70 seconds on 13 different exercise machines. If John rests less than

30 seconds between machines, he will maintain a relatively high heart rate throughout his training session, which will last about 20 minutes.

As discussed in Chapter 5, the generally accepted criteria for improving cardiovascular performance is 15–20 minutes of continuous large muscle activity at an intensity sufficient to keep the heart rate above 70 percent of maximum (Zohman, 1974). Although working one muscle group at a time does not greatly increase oxygen consumption, it does stimulate the heart to pump blood just as hard and fast as any other vigorous activity (e.g., jogging, cycling, swimming). Consequently, "short rest" strength training can improve cardiovascular performance, as evidenced by Westcott and Warren's (1985) study and Messier and Dill's (1985) study (see Chapter 5).

If one is interested only in developing muscle strength, then a longer rest between exercises is advisable. "Short rest" training utilizes more energy per minute, and the cumulative effects of fatigue become apparent during the last half of the training session. Even though a particular muscle group may be fresh, one's overall level of fatigue may prevent a maximum muscle effort on the latter exercises.

Ideally, one should perform about 20 minutes of strength training for musculoskeletal development and about 20 minutes of endurance training for cardiovascular development. However, many men and women in our busy society do not have time for a 40-minute workout three days per week. They are often hard-pressed to squeeze in a 20-minute training session before work or during their lunch break. These individuals will probably benefit most from a "short rest" strength training program. By emphasizing exercise continuity, they can complete their workout in 20 minutes, achieve a high level of musculoskeletal fitness, and attain a moderate level of cardiovascular fitness. When workout time is a limiting factor, "short rest" strength training is an efficient means for improving one's overall physical fitness.

SUMMARY OF PROGRAM DESIGN

Strength training should not be a hit-or-miss activity. Program design is a critical factor in any strength training endeavor. By incorporating the eight guidelines presented in this chapter, one can experience safe and successful strength training that increases physical fitness and reduces the risk of injury:

1. *Exercise Selection.* One exercise should be performed for each of the major muscle groups. These are the quadriceps, hamstrings, hip abductors, hip adductors, low back, abdominals, chest, upper back, shoulders, biceps, triceps, neck extensors and neck flexors.

2. *Exercise Frequency.* Because intense muscle training usually requires 48 hours recovery and rebuilding time, one should schedule three nonconsecutive workout days per week.

3. *Exercise Duration.* Each muscle group should accomplish about 60–90 seconds of continuous, high-intensity work. This corresponds to about 8–12 slow repetitions with a relatively heavy weightload.

4. *Exercise Intensity.* Intensity is the most important factor in strength development. One must use a resistance heavy enough to cause local discomfort and momentary muscle failure within 60–90 seconds of exercise.

5. *Exercise Speed.* To increase muscle tension and to decrease the risk of injury, strength training exercises should be performed slowly. Generally speaking, the lifting movement should take about two seconds and the lowering movement should take about four seconds.

6. *Exercise Range.* For maximum muscle benefit each exercise should be performed through a full range of movement, with a momentary pause in the completely contracted position.

7. *Exercise Progression.* Because physiological adaptations in muscle tissue occur slowly, resistance should not be increased abruptly. As a rule of thumb, one should increase the weightload by 5 percent when 12 repetitions can be completed in proper form.

8. *Exercise Continuity.* By taking a minimum amount of time between exercise stations, one can complete the 13 basic exercises in about 20 minutes. "Short rest" strength training is characterized by a high heart rate, a high caloric expenditure, a high strength stimulus, and a moderate cardiovascular stimulus.

Chapter Seven

Strength Training Considerations

There are several considerations that should be observed in a sensible strength training program. Although training effectiveness is foremost in everyone's mind, the most important consideration is training safety.

TRAINING SAFETY

Training safety is more than merely avoiding large-scale accidents. There are many aspects of safe training, including the prevention of sprains, strains, tears, and other soft-tissue injuries. Basically, safe training procedures can be categorized into four general areas: (1) equipment, (2) space, (3) technique, and (4) breathing.

Equipment

All training apparatus should be in good working order and periodically checked for wear. Imagine what would happen if a bench press standard collapsed with a 250-pound barbell resting on it, or if the cable snapped during heavy lat bar pull-downs. Safe equipment implies snug fitting collars that stay in place and secure the weight plates on the barbells and dumbbells during exercises. It also means barbell sleeves that revolve smoothly, pulleys that spin without sticking points, and exercise machines that operate without difficulties.

Proper adjustment for the individual exerciser, particularly on complex apparatus such as Nautilus machines, is also important. These machines are carefully designed to accommodate individual differences, such as limb lengths, and should always be repositioned for each new exerciser. The time used in making such adjustments is time well spent, since it increases the muscle training effects and decreases the possibility of injury.

Space

Most weightroom accidents are the result of training space violations. Weight training requires much more space than most people realize. Ample space is obviously needed for free weight exercises in which barbells and dumbbells are moving in every direction. Space is also needed around exercise machines, and people should give wide berth to machines that are in use. Moving pulleys, cams, cables, and weight stacks can all cause serious injuries when someone steps too near or leans against a machine carelessly. Even calisthenics-type exercises such as sit-ups, pull-ups, bar dips, and push-ups require considerable amounts of space to be executed properly.

Space is also necessary for movement among the various exercise stations. Traffic lanes must be free from machines, weight plates, and other items, as well as persons who are exercising. This means that other space must be available for placing weight plates, barbells, dumbbells, training belts, cables, towels, etc. There must also be areas of sufficient size to accommodate persons who are lifting, stretching, warming up, cooling down, conversing, or writing in their logbooks. In other words, the safe strength training facility should be spacious and uncluttered. Exercise stations should not be close together, and weight training equipment should not be left on the floor. Every item in the weightroom should have a particular place to be stored and specific places to be used. A neat and orderly strength training facility is absolutely essential for the safety of the exercisers.

Finally, space violations often result in injuries to spotters. When spotting an exercise, such as the bench press or squat, it is not necessary for the spotter to be right on top of the lifter. It is best to give the lifter plenty of room and to be ready to step in to give assistance if necessary. Even when the spotter is providing added resistance for negative work, he or she should find the most unobtrusive position and give the lifter as much room as possible to execute the exercise movements.

Technique

Accidents frequently occur as a result of improper training techniques. Persons who throw weights are more likely to injure themselves than persons who use controlled movement speeds. Persons who perform unsupported exercises, such as the standing press, have a higher risk of injury than those who do supported exercises, such as the incline press. Figure 7–1 illustrates the greater stress to the lower back imposed by unsupported, overhead pressing movements.

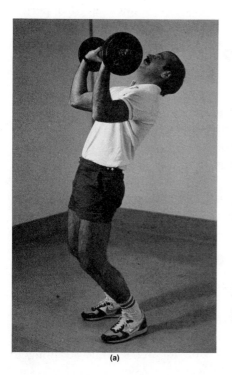
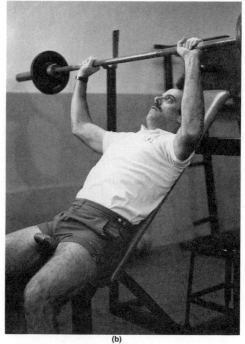

(a)   (b)

Figure 7–1a. Unsupported Standing Press; and *b.* Supported Incline Press

Many muscle injuries result from ignorance of basic biomechanical principles (see Chapter 4). For example, due to leverage factors, much less weight must be used for straight arm exercises (e.g., straight arm flies, straight arm pull-overs) than for bent arm exercises (e.g., bent arm flies, bent arm pull-overs). Unfavorable leverage arrangements are also responsible for subjecting the lower back muscles to high stress conditions in exercises such as good mornings, barbell bent rows, and stiff-legged dead lifts (see Figure 7−2).

As mentioned earlier, improper technique is an inevitable consequence of incorrect positioning on an exercise machine. It is therefore important to make the appropriate adjustments prior to executing repetitions on a mechanical exercise apparatus. For example, when using Nautilus equipment, one should make certain that the axis of rotation on the machine is directly in line with the joint being exercised.

Poor technique is frequently exhibited during attempts at personal weightlifting records. The prospect of establishing a new personal record is often sufficient incentive to cheat on a lift. Bridging on a bench press and arching on a standing curl are common maneuvers that permit heavier lifts, but place great stress on the lower back (see Figure 7−3). Perhaps, the most necessary change in the field of weight training is to place greater emphasis on the muscles and less emphasis on the weightloads. In other words, one should use the minimum amount of weight necessary to develop the maximum amount of muscle tension. This provides the safest stimulus for strength development and reduces the risk of injury due to poor form with excessive weightloads.

Due to the intensity of most weight training exercises, injuries tend to be relatively severe and often require several weeks for rehabilitation. Because many people discontinue weight training altogether after experiencing a debilitating injury, it is important to be extra safety-conscious in the weight training room. Frequent equipment checks, ample training space, and proper exercise techniques are the keys to injury-free and effective weight training programs.

Breathing During Exercise

Before experimenting with various strength training exercises, one should understand something about breathing during forceful muscular contraction. Taking a deep breath and holding it while straining to complete a repetition is a dangerous practice. The internal pressure created by breath holding coupled with the external pressure of tightly

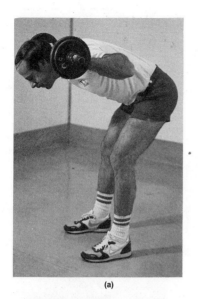

(a)

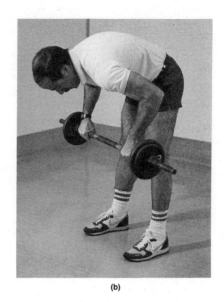

(b)

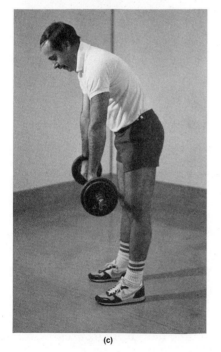

(c)

Figure 7-2a. Good Morning Exercise; *b.* Bent Row Exercise; and *c.* Stiff-Legged Dead Lift Exercise

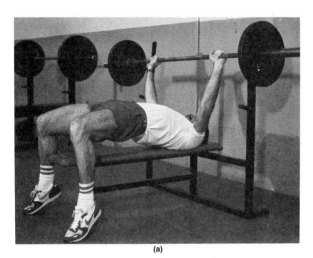

(a)

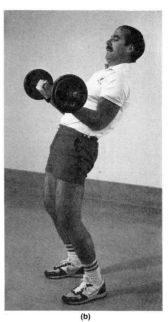

(b)

Figure 7—3a. Bench Press with Bridge; and
b. Curl with Back Bend

contracted muscles may be sufficient to limit blood flow to an area of the body. When the neck and shoulder muscles are involved, this can lead to a feeling of lightheadedness or an actual loss of consciousness.

Perhaps more important, the increased pressure in the chest area that results from holding the breath during a strenuous lifting movement can interfere with venous blood return to the heart and significantly elevate blood pressure. This undesirable reaction is known as the Valsalva Response. Consequently, the breath should never be held for a prolonged period of time when exercising with weights.

On the other hand, many exercises require the chest area to be stabilized for successful execution. Consequently, for maximum performance in exercises such as the bench press, breathing must cease momentarily. The key is to never hold the breath for more than a moment, and to breathe on every repetition.

From a physiological standpoint, the best system of breathing requires the exerciser to inhale during the lowering movement (eccentric contraction) and to exhale during the lifting movement (concentric contraction). In this manner, the internal pressure is decreased as the external pressure is increased. The opposite pattern of breathing causes the internal pressure and external pressure to increase simultaneously and should be avoided.

Most exercisers develop a breathing pattern that suits their particular training style without jeopardizing blood flow or restricting their oxygen supply. As long as one does not take deep breaths or attempt to hold the breath for more than a moment, problems should not be encountered.

TRAINING PARTNERS

Training partners are an asset to one's strength training progress. Regardless of the training program, exercise facilities, or equipment employed, a training partner fulfills a definite role. The most important thing a training partner can do is encourage the exerciser throughout the workout, and particularly during the final repetitions of each exercise set. This does not mean idle talking during the rest intervals, but genuine encouragement prior to and during each exercise bout. The solo exerciser hears only one voice, that of his or her tired muscles saying "that's enough." Persons who train together hear a second voice, that of their partners urging them to squeeze out one more repetition.

Although some persons train with more drive and singleness of purpose than others, most persons admit that they work harder when they have a training partner. Actually, partners inspire each other by alternately giving encouragement and exhibiting maximum effort during their own exercise program. This modeling effect is a significant advantage of partner training. Seeing one's partner go all-out during a training program is a great source of motivation. Outstanding coaches in all sports areas typically work their athletes in pairs or small groups for this very reason. One is less likely to merely go through the motions of a workout when a training partner is giving an unrestrained effort.

Spotters

Depending on the type of exercise being performed, training partners may be absolutely necessary. It is foolish to attempt heavy bench presses without a spotter, because an unanticipated event, such as a muscle tear, muscle spasm, or muscle cramp, could result in a serious injury. The same is true for squats, pull-overs, and any other exercise in which momentary loss of muscle control could have serious consequences.

In addition to safety considerations, the training partner can perform a valuable service in these and other exercises. For example, the exerciser may be unable to push the final repetition in the bench press past the half-way point. If the spotter gently supports a small percentage of the weightload instead of quickly lifting the bar to the standards, the exerciser will be able to force the bar upward and complete the repetition. This is referred to as a forced repetition, and is made possible by a competent training partner who gives just enough help to allow the lifter to complete the movement and more fully stress the contributing muscle groups. Forced repetitions are a standard training practice among most bodybuilders, since their goal is to continue each exercise bout to the point of maximum muscle exertion.

Along the same line, some exercisers include so-called negative work in their strength training program. It is recalled that negative work involves maximum effort against a resistance that is too great for the muscle to overcome. This is actually an eccentric contraction in which the muscle lengthens under the force of an overpowering resistance (weightload). For example, an individual may not be able to curl more than 90 pounds from the waist to the shoulders. However, the same person may slowly lower a 120-pound barbell from the shoulders to the waist by means of maximum eccentric muscle contraction. Many people believe that controlled failure (eccentric contraction) with 120 pounds provides a greater training stimulus than success (concentric contraction) with 90 pounds. For those who train in this manner, one or more partners are essential to bring the weightload to the desired starting position.

While there are several exercises in which a partner is helpful, there are others that simply cannot be done as effectively without the aid of a partner. Various stretching exercises, particularly those for the back and hamstrings, are greatly enhanced by a knowledgeable person who gently holds the partner in a stretched position, and gradually extends the range of motion. Likewise, manual resistance exercises, such as those for the neck muscles, depend on a skilled training partner who provides the right amount of resistance in the right place at the right time.

The advantage of training with one or more partners far outweighs any disadvantage, provided the partners are compatible and have similar training goals and procedures. It is not necessary for the partners to be equally matched in strength if training is done on Universal Gym or Nautilus equipment, since weightloads can be changed quickly and easily.

However, if conventional weights are utilized, the partners should not be vastly different in terms of muscle strength or much of their workout time and energy will be used for changing the weights.

TRAINING EQUIPMENT

If money and training space were no object, strength enthusiasts could choose from several types of training equipment. Although some people train with isometric exercises, most strength training equipment falls into two categories: isokinetics and isotonics.

The basic difference between isokinetic exercise and isotonic exercise may be described as follows. With isokinetic exercise, the muscle effort determines the resistance. In other words, more muscle effort produces more resistance and less muscle effort produces less resistance. With isotonic exercise, the resistance determines the muscle effort. In other words, more resistance produces more muscle effort and less resistance produces less muscle effort.

Isokinetic Equipment

To better understand the isokinetic principle of training, stand in the shallow end of a swimming pool and move your hand against the water. When you apply little force, your hand meets little resistance. When you apply greater force, your hand meets greater resistance.

There are many types of isokinetic strength training devices available for commercial use. These include Cybex machines, Hydra-Fitness machines, and Mini-Gym apparatus.

Barbells and Dumbbells

Barbells and dumbbells have been basic to strength training programs for years, and are still the most familiar and widely used type of exercise equipment (see Figure 7—4). Between barbells, designed for two-handed lifts, and dumbbells, designed for one-handed lifts, a number of exercises can be performed with free weights. As the name implies, free weights are not attached to any fixtures or machines and can be manipulated by the exerciser in any way desired.

Free weights can be used for both concentric contractions (positive work) and eccentric contractions (negative work). However, because the

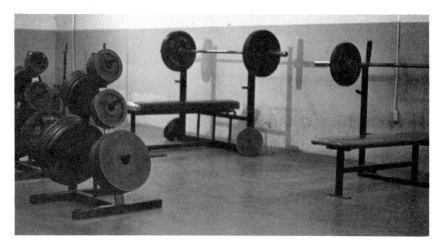

Figure 7−4. Barbell Equipment

muscles and bones of the body function as lever systems, a given barbell may feel lighter in one position and heavier in another position. Every free weight exercise has a sticking point, the place in the range of movement at which the mechanical factors are least favorable and the greatest amount of muscle force is required. It is the point where the exerciser succeeds or fails in making the lift.

For example, in the bench press exercise the sticking point is near the chest, as illustrated in Figure 7−5. Greater muscular effort is required at this point in the bench press movement than at any other, due to the mechanical factors involved. In terms of training efficiency, the heaviest barbell one can bench press (1RM weightload) actually produces maximum muscular stress at only one point in the entire range of movement. Once the barbell is pressed beyond the sticking point, less muscular effort is required to complete the lift, because the body's lever arrangements become more favorable. Consequently, movements that incorporate a fixed resistance necessarily produce different levels of muscle stress at different points in the range of movement. For further information on barbells and dumbbells see Appendix A.

Universal Gym Equipment

Universal Gym equipment has popularized traditional weight training by making it safe, convenient, space efficient, and time efficient (see Figure 7−6). The Universal Gym includes a number of exercise stations at

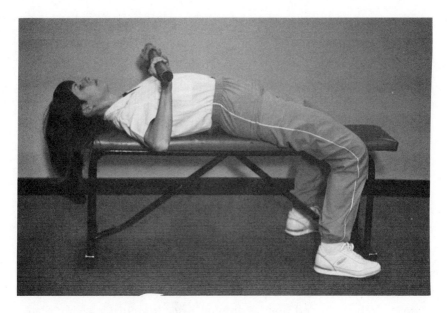

Figure 7-5. Bench Press Sticking Point

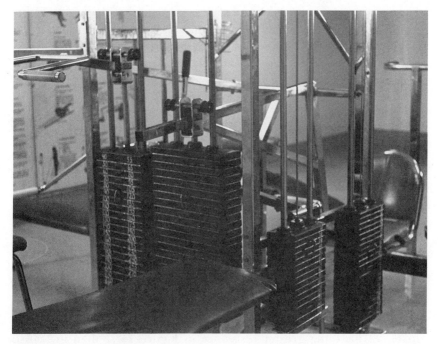

Figure 7-6. Universal Gym Equipment

which smooth-running weight stacks are lifted by lever and pulley attachments. Because the weights travel on fixed tracks away from the exerciser, spotters are not necessary, and the possibility of being injured by a falling weight is greatly reduced.

The Universal Gym, although a relatively heavy piece of equipment, can be easily moved from place to place by a single person. Once located, the Universal Gym becomes a one-stop training center, with stations for bench presses, lat bar pull-downs, overhead presses, curls, triceps pressdowns, upright rows, seated rows, shoulder shrugs, leg presses, toe raises, sit-ups, back extensions, pull-ups, hanging knee-ups, dips, and a variety of improvised exercises. An additional piece of Universal Gym equipment enables the exerciser to perform leg extensions, leg curls, forearm exercises, and neck exercises.

Both pieces of Universal Gym equipment can be safely and comfortably placed in a small room or in a corner of the regular weight training facility. The stations are designed to minimize space requirements and yet permit several persons to exercise concurrently. Because the Universal Gym is a self-contained unit, additional space for storing weight plates, bars, and exercise attachments is unnecessary.

Another aspect of the Universal Gym that has made it a popular training apparatus is the quick and effortless method of changing weightloads. By simply removing and reinserting a steel pin, one can change the exercise weightload by several hundred pounds, a process that would require considerable time and effort with free weights. Time is also saved by the proximity of the various exercise stations to each other. The Universal Gym is well-suited for persons who prefer to do a sequence of different exercises with as little rest between exercises as possible.

Until recently, the numerous exercise stations, the small space requirements, and the safe and easily adjusted weight stacks were the key features of Universal Gym equipment. However, the newer Universal Gym models now provide automatically variable resistance at some of the exercise stations, which has certain advantages over fixed resistance training.

As previously indicated, muscles are capable of handling more weight at some points in the range of movement than others due to leverage factors. In the bench press exercise, for example, the muscles can handle progressively more weight as the arms become more fully extended. In other words, the muscles are capable of overcoming more resistance in Figure 7–7b than in Figure 7–7a. Similarly, the muscles are capable of handling greater resistance in Figure 7–7c than in Figure 7–7b.

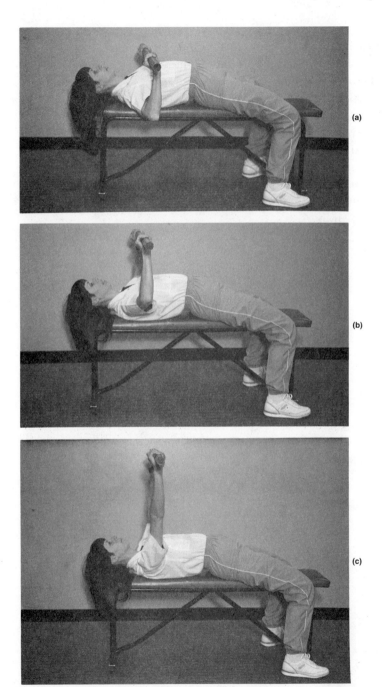

Figure 7−7a. Bench Press, Poor Leverage; *b.* Bench Press, Moderate Leverage; and *c.* Bench Press, Good Leverage

With this in mind, the new Universal Gym bench press station automatically increases the resistance as the arms are extended. This is accomplished by moving the position of the resistance along the lifting lever (see Figure 7−8). Thus, leverage changes in the machine require greater effective muscle force. Although this method of varying the exercise resistance does not perfectly accommodate the changes in effective muscle strength, it is certainly a step in the right direction. Because the muscles are forced to work at closer to maximum levels through a greater portion of the exercise movement, variable resistance training may be a more efficient means of strength development than fixed resistance training. For further information on Universal Gym equipment, see Appendix A.

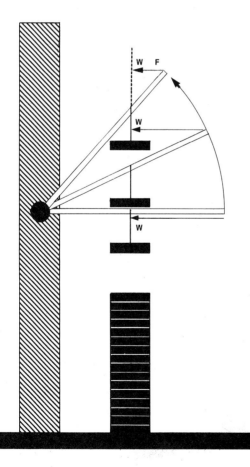

Figure 7−8. Schematic diagram illustrating how automatically variable resistance can be provided by a moving resistance on the lifting lever. As the lever is moved upward, the distance between the applied force (F) and the weightload (W) decreases, increasing the effective resistance.

Nautilus Equipment

Perhaps the most significant advancements in the field of strength training have been the introduction of Nautilus training principles and Nautilus training equipment (see Figure 7–9). Nautilus machines have four features that enhance the attainment of muscle isolation, stress intensification, and personal motivation. These are: (1) supportive structure, (2) rotary movement, (3) direct resistance, and (4) automatically variable resistance.

Supportive Structure. Muscle isolation is enhanced when exercises are performed from a supported position. When one is sitting or lying on a machine, the posture muscles are relaxed, and the effort is focused on the target muscle groups.

For example, when one performs a standing curl, the muscles of the legs and back must contract isometrically to maintain erect posture and balance. On the other hand, the Nautilus Multi-Curl Machine allows the exerciser to work from a supported position with minimum involvement of the leg and back muscles.

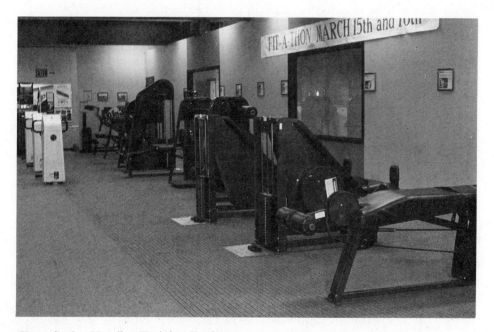

Figure 7–9. Nautilus Training Equipment

In addition to increased muscle isolation, supportive structure provides decreased risk of injury. When training in a standing position, one is more likely to use and misuse the leg and trunk muscles, especially during the final repetitions.

Rotary Movement. Almost all movements in the human body involve the rotation of a bone about a joint axis. Although every muscle pulls in a straight line, the resulting joint movement is circular. Movements about the ankle, knee, hip, shoulder, elbow and wrist are of a rotary nature. Only when an exercise involves more than one joint can a linear movement be produced.

This being the case, rotary movements permit muscle isolation, and linear movements prohibit muscle isolation. Most barbell and Universal Gym exercises require linear movements (e.g., squats, presses, and pull-downs). On the other hand, most Nautilus machines are designed to apply resistance in a rotary movement, with the machine axis of rotation aligned with the joint axis of rotation.

Rotary movements enhance both muscle isolation and stress intensification. In a linear movement, the resistance is directly opposed to the muscle force in only one position, when the movement arm is at a right angle to the resistive force. In a rotary movement, the resistance is directly opposed to the muscle force in every position, because the movement arm is always at a right angle to the resistive force.

For example, the latissimus muscles move the upper arms from a position overhead to a position against the sides. With conventional barbells, the most common exercise for the latissimus muscles is bent rowing. Bent rowing involves a restricted range of joint motion (about 90 degrees) and linear movement of the barbell (see Figures 6−6 and 6−7).

With Universal Gym equipment, the usual exercise for the latissimus muscles is the lat bar pull-down. Although lat bar pull-downs provide a greater range of motion than bent rowing (approximately 180 degrees), they too involve only linear movement of the lat bar and cable (see Figures 6−8 and 6−9).

The Nautilus pull-over machine provides both an extended range of motion (over 240 degrees) and rotary movement about the shoulder joint (see Figure 7−10). In this exercise, both the upper arms and the resistance lever move through the same circular path as they rotate around the shoulder axis. This rotary action puts the resistive force in direct opposition to the movement force through the entire range of motion. The bent-row and the lat bar pull-down, on the other hand,

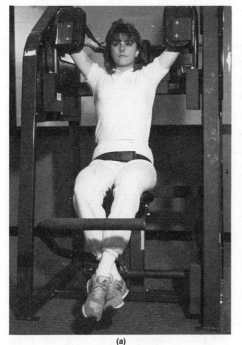 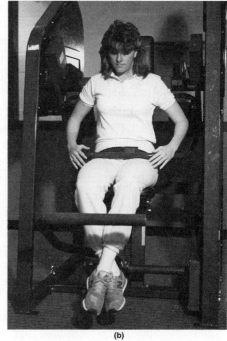

(a)   (b)

Figure 7–10a. Nautilus Pull-over Start; and *b.* Nautilus Pull-over Finish

provide resistance only in the vertical plane. In these exercises, the resistive force is in direct opposition to the movement force for a relatively small segment of the exercise movement (i.e., when the upper arms are approximately parallel to the floor). It is suggested that rotary movement exercises provide a safer and more efficient means of strength development than exercises that provide resistance in only one plane.

   Direct Resistance. Direct resistance implies that the resistive force is applied to the same body segment to which the movement force is applied. For example, the latissimus muscles are attached to the upper arm, and their function is to pull the upper arms toward the sides of the body. In order to provide direct resistance to the latissimus muscles, the resistive force must be applied to the upper arms.

   As illustrated in Figures 6–6 and 6–7, this is not the case with conventional barbell training. The resistance in the bent row exercise is applied to the lower arms (hands) rather than to the upper arms. Execution of the exercise involves the wrist joint, elbow joint, and shoulder joint.

Stated differently, the bent row exercise cannot be completed without the forearm muscles and upper arm muscles. Consequently, when these smaller muscles become fatigued, the bent rows must be discontinued even though the larger latissimus muscles have not been fully stressed.

A similar situation exists with the lat bar pull-downs on the Universal Gym (see Figures 6–8 and 6–9). The resistance is applied to the lower arms (hands) rather than to the upper arms. As with bent rows, execution of lat bar pull-downs involves the wrist joint, elbow joint, and shoulder joint. When the weaker arm muscles become fatigued, the lat bar pull-downs must be discontinued, even though the stronger latissimus muscles have not been fully stressed.

One of the unique features of the Nautilus pull-over machine is that the resistance is applied directly to the upper arm. In other words, both the movement force provided by the latissimus muscles and the movement resistance provided by the weight stack act upon the same body part. Because no assisting muscle groups are involved, the exercise can and should be continued until the latissimus muscles become completely fatigued.

Direct resistance is a practical application of the Principle of Training Specificity. Exercises that involve more than one muscle group (two joint movements) tend to stress the smaller muscle groups to a greater degree than the larger muscle group. If the larger muscle group is prevented from being fully stressed, it is not likely to develop strength as efficiently as it could. For this reason, Nautilus has designed direct resistance exercise machines for the muscles that move the upper arms, namely the latissimus muscles, chest muscles, and shoulder muscles. Direct resistance exercises should continue until the target muscles become exhausted, which should in turn stimulate desirable strength adaptations.

Variable Resistance. Because changes in lever arrangements are basic to human movement, there are stronger positions and weaker positions in every range of joint movement. Consequently, a barbell that provides maximum resistance at the weakest point in an exercise movement offers less than maximum resistance at all other points in the movement. As previously discussed, Universal Gym equipment incorporates a lever arm with a movable resistance to compensate for leverage changes in the body. While this means of producing variable resistance works reasonably well with the bench press exercise, it is not applicable to exercises such as lat bar pull-downs, curls, triceps press-downs, rows, leg curls, leg extensions, and other exercises that do not involve a horizontal lever arm.

The variable resistance approach developed by Nautilus utilizes an oval-shaped cam to automatically change the resistance throughout the range of movement. The cam is designed around the ideal strength curve (leverage changes) for a particular exercise. The strength curve represents the changes in effective muscle strength experienced during a given full-range movement. For example, the cam provides greater resistance during the middle part of the biceps curl than during the first part of the biceps curl, which is consistent with the strength curve for this particular arm movement. If a circular wheel were used, the distance from the axis of rotation to the point where the chain leaves the wheel would not change, the mechanics of the system would not be altered, and the resistance would stay the same throughout the entire range of movement (see Figure 7−11). However, the oval shape of the Nautilus cam changes the distance from the axis of rotation to the point where the chain leaves the cam. This changes the mechanics of the system and produces a corresponding variation in resistance throughout the movement range (see Figure 7−12). More specifically, as the distance from the axis of rotation to the chain increases, the resistance increases. Conversely, as the distance from the axis of rotation to the chain decreases, the resistance decreases.

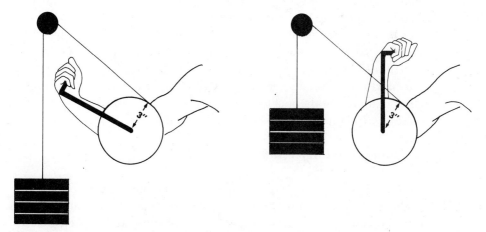

Figure 7−11. A circular wheel does not change the distance from the axis of rotation to the chain at the point where it leaves the wheel. The resistance therefore remains the same through the entire range of movement.

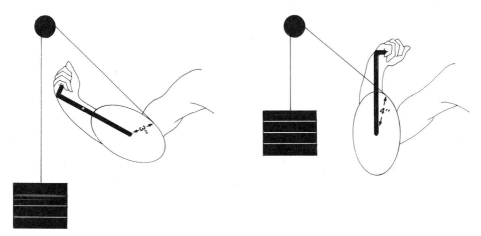

Figure 7—12.   An oval-shaped cam changes the distance from the axis of rotation to the chain at the point where it leaves the cam. This changes the mechanical advantage and varies the resistance accordingly throughout the range of movement.

Although the shape of the Nautilus cam is based on the ideal strength curve for each of the exercise movements, it produces a relatively constant stress on the muscles throughout the range of motion. That is, the resistance does not feel lighter in some positions than in others. The use of cams designed for specific movement patterns appears to be both an effective and practical means of providing automatically variable resistance. Variable resistance training may be a more efficient method of strength development than fixed resistance training because it requires near-maximum muscular effort through the entire range of movement, rather than only at the sticking point. For further information on Nautilus Strength Training Machines, see Appendix A.

Equipment Selection

There is no question that people have developed great strength and excellent physiques with barbell training, Universal Gym training, and Nautilus training, as well as with isokinetic training and isometric training. As long as the basic principles of strength development are followed, most persons will make progress towards their desired training objectives. Although time and money are major factors in the choice of training equipment, the most important aspect of any strength training program is personal satisfaction.

One aspect of personal satisfaction is training motivation. The visible weightstack utilized in isotonic training (e.g., barbells, Universal Gym, Nautilus) is an excellent source of feedback and reinforcement. Most people like to see tangible evidence of their exercise efforts, and additional weight plates clearly indicate performance progress.

Another important factor in strength training is the eccentric contraction. Controlled lowering of a weight provides a critical stimulus for muscle development. Because isokinetic devices do not permit eccentric muscle contractions, isotonic training is more advantageous in this regard.

In the final analysis, it is suggested that strength development is facilitated by the following training factors: (1) supportive structure, (2) rotary movement, (3) direct resistance, (4) automatically variable resistance, (5) visible weightstack, and (6) eccentric contractions.

ACTIVITY INTEGRATION

Many fitness enthusiasts perform other physical activities in addition to strength training. Some prefer endurance activities such as jogging, cycling, swimming, cross-country skiing, canoeing, and rowing. Others participate in sports activities such as soccer, basketball, tennis, racquetball, volleyball, and softball. Still others enjoy recreational activities such as walking, hiking, golf, horseback riding, and dancing.

While there is nothing wrong with performing a variety of physical activities, it is necessary to properly integrate these activities to avoid overtraining. For example, it would be unrealistic to attempt a hard strength workout following a day of cross-country skiing.

It is generally accepted that high-intensity strength training requires about 48 hours between sessions for muscle repair and rebuilding. Any strength-related activity performed during that time is likely to interfere with muscle recovery. However, strenuous endurance activity may also delay the rebuilding process, since more energy stores must be replenished.

Consider the person who wants to combine strength training and endurance training. It is recommended that every other day be a hard training day with an easy training day in between. That is, one should take a hard strength workout and a hard endurance workout on the same day. The following day should be a recovery day, with no strength training and only easy endurance training. Depending on the training intensity, two recovery days may be necessary before the next hard workout.

One research study (Westcott, 1986g) indicates that the activity order may affect performance. The subjects in this study attempted to perform two identical workouts. In one session, they first did a specific strength program (Nautilus), rested five minutes, and then did a specific endurance program (computerized cycle ergometer). In another session they first did the endurance program, rested five minutes, and then did the strength program.

As illustrated in Figures 7–13 and 7–14, the activity order had a greater influence on endurance performance than on strength performance. That is, the strength performance was essentially the same in both training sessions. However, the endurance performance produced a higher heart rate response when it followed the strength workout.

Based on these findings, it would appear that endurance training

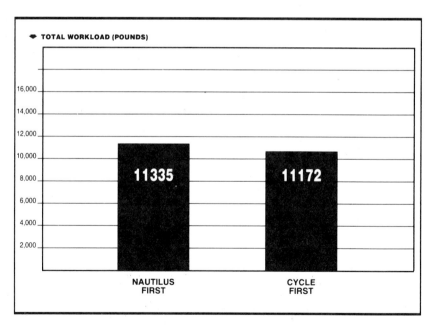

Figure 7–13.   Effect of Activity Order on Strength Performance During Nautilus Workout

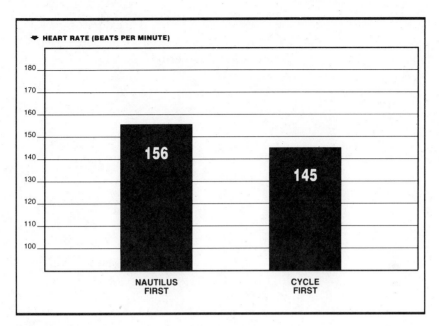

Figure 7-14. Effect of Activity Order on Endurance Performance During Cycle Ergometer Workout

should precede strength training when both workouts are taken close together. However, it is suggested that better results may be obtained by resting four to six hours between the endurance workout and the strength workout. For example, one could take a hard endurance workout before work and a hard strength workout during the lunch hour. This provides a reasonable buffer zone between the two workouts without intruding too much into the rebuilding period.

Highly skilled activities such as tennis, soccer, basketball, and volley-ball should not be performed immediately after high-intensity strength training. The forceful muscle contractions, blood infusion, and local muscle fatigue seem to have an adverse affect on neuromuscular coordination for a short period of time. Like endurance training, it is recommended that these sports activities be performed four to six hours after the strength workout.

Low-intensity activities such as walking, golf, and bowling require little recovery energy and may be performed at one's discretion. However, regardless of one's physical condition, it is a good policy to follow a hard day–easy day training program. Remember that exercise is merely a stimulus for physical improvement. The beneficial adaptations take place only during the recovery and rebuilding period.

Chapter Eight

Strength Training Exercises

The three keys to successful strength training are muscle isolation, stress intensification, and personal motivation. With few exceptions, the exercises presented in this chapter meet these criteria. Most of the exercises emphasize a specific muscle group, facilitate stress intensification, and foster personal motivation.

The exercises are presented under the following categories: (1) quadriceps, (2) hamstrings, (3) hip adductors, (4) hip abductors, (5) low back, (6) abdominals, (7) chest, (8) upper back, (9) shoulders, (10) triceps, (11) biceps, (12) neck flexors, (13) neck extensors, (14) calves, (15) forearms, and (16) trapezius. Each exercise should be performed slowly and safely through a full-range of movement. The weightload should permit 8 to 12 repetitions in good form, and the exerciser should inhale and exhale during every repetition.

QUADRICEPS

The quadriceps are one of the largest and strongest muscle groups in the human body. The quadriceps are responsible for extending the knee and for flexing the hip. There are three basic exercises for strengthening the quadriceps muscles.

Leg Extension

As illustrated in Figure 8–1, the leg extension is a rotary exercise that largely isolates the quadriceps muscles.

Technical Points:
1. Sit on seat and align knee joint with machine axis of rotation.
2. Use additional pad for back support if necessary.
3. Fasten seat belt.
4. Place hands on handgrips.
5. Place ankles in neutral position behind lever arm.
6. Slowly lift lever arm until the quadriceps are fully contracted and hold momentarily.

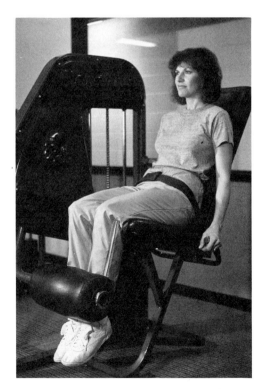

Figure 8–1. Leg Extension

7. Slowly lower lever arm until plates almost touch weightstack, and repeat.

Note: By not allowing the plates to rest on the weightstack, muscle tension is maintained throughout the exercise set.

Barbell Squat

As illustrated in Figure 8−2, the Barbell Squat is a linear exercise that emphasizes the quadriceps muscles.

Technical Points:
1. Place barbell across the upper back, and lift it off the supporting rack.
2. Hands should be wide spaced, and feet should be shoulder width apart.

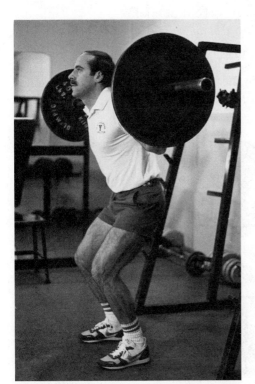

Figure 8−2. Barbell Squat

3. Slowly lower the body until the thighs are approximately parallel to the floor.
4. Slowly raise the body to a standing position and repeat.
5. Keep the head up and the back straight throughout the exercise.

Note: It is important to incorporate a spotter or a safety rack when performing barbell squats.

Duo-Squat

As illustrated in Figure 8−3, the duo-squat is a linear exercise that emphasizes the quadriceps muscles.

Technical Points:
1. Lie on decline seat with head supported on pad.
2. Place both feet on foot pedals simultaneously.
3. Place hands on handgrips.
4. Extend both legs to near lockout position.
5. At this position the lever arms should touch the restraining bolts, thereby assuring proper cam function. If this does not occur, the seat must be readjusted.
6. Maintain the left leg in the near lockout position and bring the right leg slowly towards the chest.

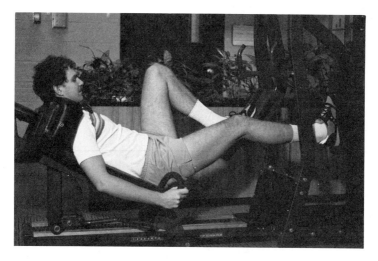

Figure 8−3.   Duo-Squat

7. Extend the right leg slowly to the near lockout position.
8. Maintain the right leg in the near lockout position and bring the left leg slowly towards the chest.
9. Extend the left leg slowly to the near lockout position.
10. Continue to alternate legs until no more repetitions can be performed, and slowly lower plates to weightstack.

Note: An alternative method of performing the duo-squat is to incorporate the infimetric bar and work one leg against the other while holding the plates in the top position.

HAMSTRINGS

The hamstrings perform the opposite movements to the quadriceps. They are responsible for knee flexion and hip extension. The basic exercise for strengthening the hamstrings is the leg curl.

Leg Curl

As shown in Figure 8–4, the leg curl is a rotary exercise that largely isolates the hamstring muscles.

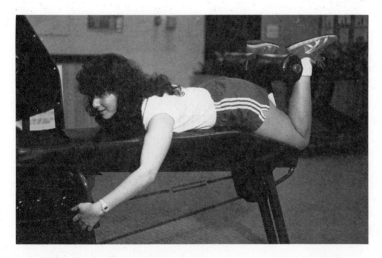

Figure 8–4. Leg Curl

Technical Points:
1. Lie on seat and align knee joint with machine axis of rotation.
2. Place hands on handgrips.
3. Place ankles in neutral position behind lever arm.
4. Slowly lift lever arm until the hamstrings are fully contracted and hold momentarily.
5. Slowly lower lever arm until plates almost touch weightstack and repeat.

Note: For complete contraction of the hamstring muscles, the hips must raise slightly off the support pad.

HIP ADDUCTORS

The hip adductor muscles move the legs sideways towards the midline of the body. The hip adductor exercise seems to best isolate this muscle group.

Hip Adductor

As shown in Figure 8–5, the hip adductor is a rotary exercise in which the hip joint is the axis of rotation.

Technical Points:
1. Sit on seat with back fully supported.
2. Fasten seat belt.
3. Place hands on handgrips.
4. Place legs outside knee and ankle pads.
5. Slowly move legs together and hold momentarily in final position.
6. Slowly move legs apart until comfortably stretched and repeat.

Note: Assistance may be necessary to place the legs into the starting position.

HIP ABDUCTORS

The hip abductor muscles are antagonistic to the hip adductor muscles. They move the legs sideways, away from the midline of the body.

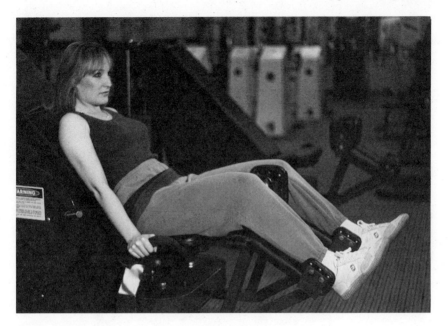

Figure 8–5. Hip Adductor

The hip abductor exercise seems most effective for isolating this muscle group.

Hip Abductor

As presented in Figure 8–6, the hip abductor is a rotary exercise in which the hip joint is the axis of rotation.

Technical Points:
1. Sit on seat.
2. Fasten seat belt.
3. Place hands on handgrips.
4. Place legs inside knee and ankle pads.
5. Slowly move legs apart and hold momentarily in final position.
6. Slowly move legs together until plates almost touch weightstack, and repeat.

Note: It is important to attain a full range of movement in this exercise.

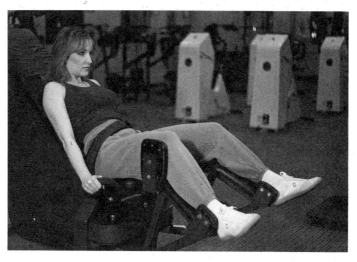

Figure 8−6.   Hip Abductor

LOW BACK

The back extensors are the strongest muscles in the body. They are powerfully involved in back extension and hip extension. The back extension exercise works these muscles through a large movement range.

Back Extension

As illustrated in Figure 8−7, the back extension is a rotary exercise that emphasizes the low back muscles.

Technical Points:
1. Sit on seat in front of lever arm with feet evenly spaced on floor grid.
2. Fasten seat belt and secure thigh pads.
3. Fold arms across chest and keep head in neutral position.
4. Slowly push lever arm backwards to extended position and pause momentarily.
5. Return slowly until plates almost touch weightstack and repeat.

Note: It is important to perform all lower back movements slowly.

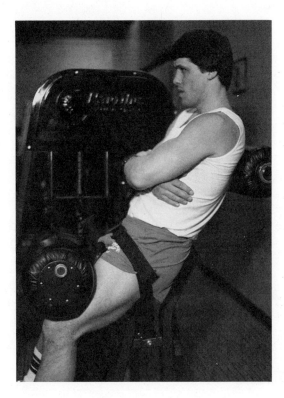

Figure 8−7. Back Extension

ABDOMINALS

The abdominal muscles are responsible for trunk flexion and assist with hip flexion. The abdominal curl addresses both of these functions. The oblique muscle located on either side of the abdominals provide lateral movement about the midsection. The rotary torso exercise largely isolates the oblique muscles.

Abdominal Curl

As shown in Figure 8−8, the abdominal curl is a rotary exercise that emphasizes the abdominal muscles.

Technical Points:
1. Sit on seat behind torso pads, with feet secured beneath foot rollers.

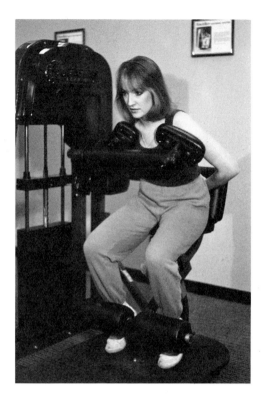

Figure 8–8.   Abdominal Curl

2. Place hands behind back.
3. Slowly push lever arm forward until parallel with floor, and pause momentarily.
4. Return slowly until plates almost touch weightstack, and repeat.

Note: The seat should be adjusted so that the top of the torso pads and the top of the shoulders are even.

Rotary Torso

As illustrated in Figures 8–9 and 8–10, the rotary torso is a rotary exercise performed in two parts.

Technical Points:
1. Sit on seat with back straight and in line with machine axis of rotation.

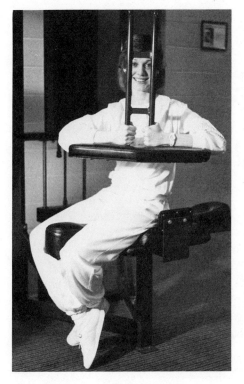

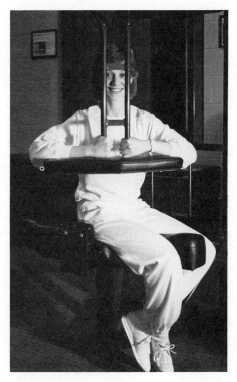

Figure 8−9.   Rotary Torso Right   ***Figure 8−10.***   Rotary Torso Left

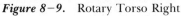

2. Place forearms and hands on movement arm.
3. Bring movement arm to neutral position directly in front of face.
4. With head, shoulders, and torso in a fixed position, turn slowly towards the weightstack, about 45 degrees past the neutral position.
5. After a momentary pause, turn slowly away from the weight- stack, about 45 degrees past the neutral position.
6. Repeat this 90 degree movement pattern until fatigued and slowly return plates to weightstack.
7. Change seat position to face opposite direction and repeat the above procedures.

Note: Because the oblique muscles have a limited range of motion, it is important to restrict the exercise movement to 45 degrees either side of the neutral position.

CHEST

The chest muscles move the upper arms forwards, downwards, and diagonally across the torso. The following four exercises are effective for strengthening the chest muscles.

10-Degree Chest

As presented in Figure 8–11, the 10-degree chest is a rotary exercise that emphasizes the chest muscles.

Technical Points:
1. Lie on seat with feet on floor, foot rest, or stool.
2. Place upper arms under roller pads.
3. Slowly raise roller pads until they meet directly above chest and hold momentarily.
4. Slowly lower roller pads until plates almost touch weightstack and repeat.

Note: The head should remain on the seat throughout the exercise.

Chest Cross

As illustrated in Figure 8–12, the chest cross is a rotary exercise that emphasizes the chest muscles.

Technical Points:
1. Sit on seat, and align shoulder joints with machine axes of rotation.
2. Reposition seat or use additional pad as necessary.
3. Fasten seat belt.
4. Place forearms against arm pads, with hands lightly resting on handles and upper arms parallel to floor.
5. Slowly bring arm pads together in front of face and hold momentarily.
6. Slowly move arm pads apart until plates almost touch weightstack and repeat.

Note: The head and shoulders should remain on the seat throughout the exercise.

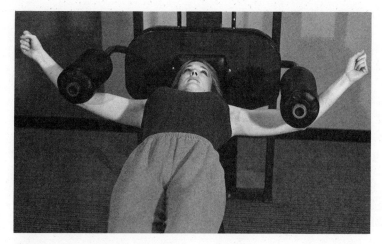

Figure 8−11.   10-Degree Chest

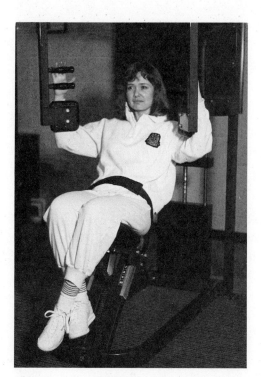

Figure 8−12.   Chest Cross

Barbell Bench Press

As shown in Figure 8–13, the barbell bench press is a linear exercise that emphasizes the chest muscles.

Technical Points:
1. Lie on bench with feet on floor.
2. Grasp barbell with hands slightly more than shoulder width apart.
3. Lift barbell from standards and hold in lockout position above chest.
4. Slowly lower barbell to chest.
5. Slowly press barbell up to lockout position and repeat.

Note: The head, shoulders, and hips should remain on the bench throughout the exercise.

Bar Dip

As presented in Figure 8–14, the bar dip is a linear exercise that emphasizes the chest muscles.

Technical Points:
1. Begin exercise with arms fully extended in lockout position.
2. Slowly lower body until upper arms are parallel to floor.
3. Slowly press body upwards until arms are fully extended and repeat.

Note: This exercise should be performed with a straight body and a neutral head position. Resistance can be increased by attaching the weightbelt. Persons unable to press their bodyweight should lower slowly and walk back up to the starting position.

UPPER BACK

The upper back includes a number of large muscle groups that move the arms backwards and downwards. The following five exercises are useful for strengthening the upper back muscles.

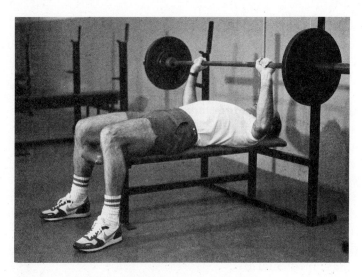

Figure 8—13. Barbell Bench Press

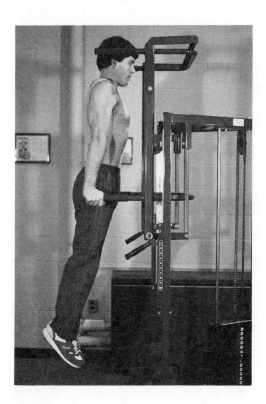

Figure 8—14. Bar Dip

Super Pull-over

As illustrated in Figure 8−15, the super pull-over is a rotary exercise that emphasizes the upper back muscles.

Technical Points:
1. Sit on seat and align shoulder joints with machine axes of rotation.
2. Reposition seat or use additional pad as necessary.
3. Fasten seat belt.
4. Press foot lever to bring arm pads into position.
5. Place upper arms against arm pads, and grip movement bar lightly with hands.
6. Slowly bring movement bar downward until it contacts seat belt and pause momentarily.
7. Slowly bring movement bar upward until shoulders are comfortably stretched and repeat.

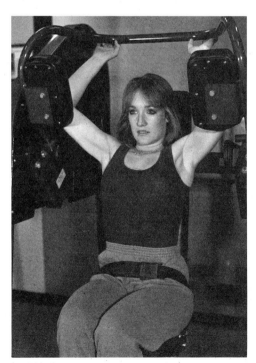

Figure 8−15.   Super Pull-Over

8. After final repetition, press foot lever to disengage arms and lower plates to weightstack.

Note: The downward movement should be accompanied by a slight trunk flexion to maintain support behind the lower back. The major movement force should come from the upper arms rather than from the hands.

Rowing Torso

As shown in Figure 8–16, the rowing torso is a rotary exercise that emphasizes the upper back muscles.

Technical Points:
1. Sit on seat with enough pads to make a snug fit.
2. Place upper arms inside roller pads, parallel to floor.

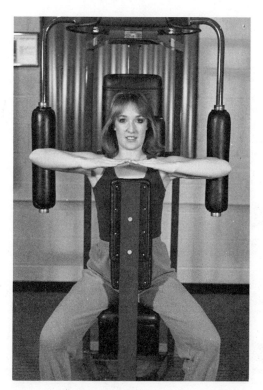

Figure 8–16. Rowing Torso

3. Slowly move roller pads backward as far as possible and hold momentarily.
4. Slowly move roller pads forward until plates almost touch weightstack and repeat.

Note: Back should remain straight, and elbows should remain high throughout this exercise.

Pull-Up

As presented in Figure 8−17, the pull-up is a linear exercise that emphasizes the upper back muscles.

Technical Points:
1. Begin exercise with hands about shoulder width apart and with arms fully extended.

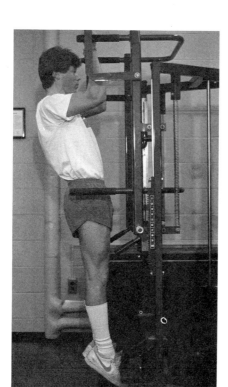

Figure 8−17.   Pull-Up

2. Slowly lift body until chin is well above bar and hold momentarily.
3. Slowly lower body to fully extended position and repeat.

Note: This exercise should be performed with a relatively straight body and a neutral head position. Resistance can be increased by attaching the weightbelt. Persons unable to lift their bodyweight should lower slowly and walk back up to the starting position.

Pull-Down

As illustrated in Figure 8−18, the pull-down is a linear exercise that emphasizes the upper back muscles.

Technical Points:
1. Sit on seat with upper legs secured.
2. Grasp bar with hands about shoulder width apart, palms facing.
3. Pull bar downward slowly and hold momentarily at chest level.
4. Slowly return bar to arm extended position and repeat.

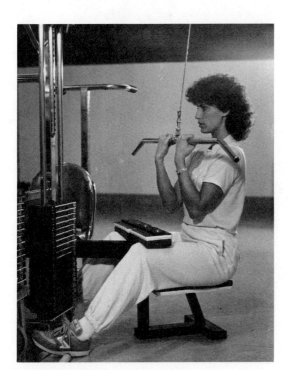

Figure 8−18.   Pull-Down

Note: Underhand grip permits greater movement range and places biceps in better mechanical position.

Dumbbell Rowing

As shown in Figure 8–19, dumbbell rowing is a linear exercise that stresses the upper back muscles.

Technical Points:
1. Bend at waist and place one hand on bench.
2. Grip dumbbell with other hand at full arm extension.
3. Slowly lift dumbbell to shoulder and hold momentarily.
4. Slowly lower dumbbell to full arm extension and repeat.

Note: It is important to place one hand on bench to support upper body and reduce stress on lower back.

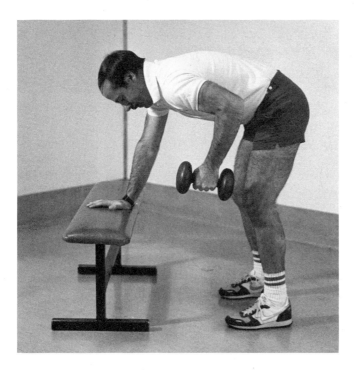

Figure 8–19. Dumbbell Rowing

SHOULDERS

The shoulder muscles are involved in forward, backward, and up-ward movements of the arms. The following three exercises emphasize the shoulder muscles.

Lateral Raise

As presented in Figure 8—20, the lateral raise is a rotary exercise that largely isolates the shoulder muscles.

Technical Points:
1. Sit on seat and align shoulder joints with machine axes of ro-tation.
2. Reposition seat or use additional pad as necessary.
3. Fasten seat belt.

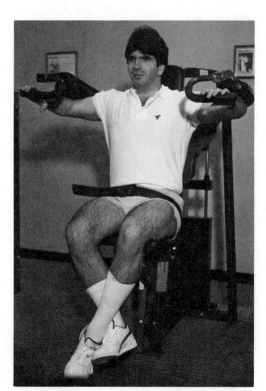

Figure 8—20.   Lateral Raise

4. Place upper arms against arm pads and grip handles loosely.
5. Slowly lift arm pads to shoulder level and hold momentarily.
6. Slowly lower arm pads until arms almost touch sides and repeat.

Note: Keep back straight and head in neutral position throughout the exercise. By not letting arms rest on sides, constant tension is maintained on shoulder muscles.

Barbell Upright Row

As presented in Figure 8−21, the Barbell Upright Row is a linear exercise that emphasizes the shoulder muscles.

Technical Points:
1. Hold bar with a close, overhand grip.

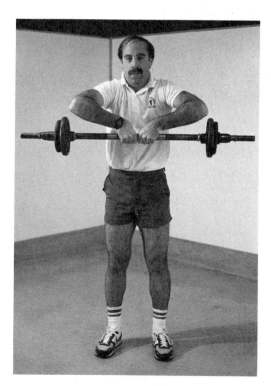

Figure 8−21. Barbell Upright Row

2. Slowly lift bar to chin with elbows leading and hold momentarily.
3. Slowly lower bar to full arm extension and repeat.

Note: Head and torso should remain erect throughout this exercise.

Barbell Incline Press

As illustrated in Figure 8–22, the barbell incline press is a linear exercise that emphasizes the shoulder muscles.

Technical Points:
1. Sit on bench with feet on floor.
2. Grasp barbell with hands slightly more than shoulder width apart.
3. Lift barbell from standards and hold in lockout position above face.

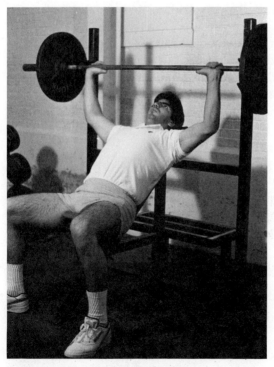

Figure 8–22.   Barbell Incline Press

4. Slowly lower barbell to upper chest.
5. Slowly press barbell upward to lockout position and repeat.

Note: The head, shoulders, and hips should remain on the bench throughout the exercise.

TRICEPS

The triceps muscles extend the elbows. The following three exercises are useful for strengthening the triceps.

Triceps Extension

As shown in Figure 8–23, the triceps extension is a rotary exercise that largely isolates the triceps muscles.

Technical Points:
1. Sit on seat and place elbows on pad in line with machine axes of rotation.
2. Reposition seat or use additional pads as necessary.
3. Place side of hands on hand pads.
4. Slowly press hand pads forward until arms are fully extended and hold momentarily.
5. Slowly return hand pads until arms are comfortably flexed and repeat.

Note: It is important to keep the elbows on the elbow pad at all times during the exercise. Shoulders should be parallel or slightly lower than elbows. An alternative method for performing the triceps extension is to incorporate the infimetric bar and work one arm against the other while holding the plates in the top position (see Figure 8–24).

Triceps Press-Down

As illustrated in Figure 8-25, the triceps press-down is a linear exercise that emphasizes the triceps muscles.

Technical Points:
1. Stand in front of press-down apparatus and hold bar with a close, overhand grip.

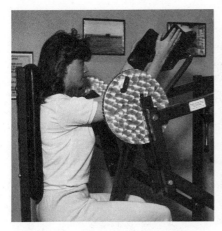 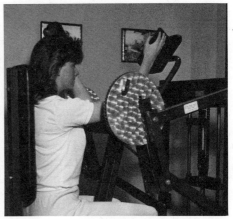

Figure 8—23. Triceps Extension   ***Figure 8—24.*** Triceps Extension Infimetric Bar

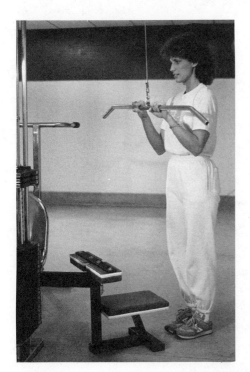

Figure 8—25. Triceps Press-Down

2. Bring bar to starting position under chin, with elbows firmly against the sides.
3. Slowly press bar downwards until arms are fully extended.
4. Slowly return bar to starting position and repeat.

Note: It is important to keep the torso erect and the elbows stabilized against the sides throughout the exercise.

Bar Dip

As shown in Figure 8–26, the bar dip is a linear exercise that emphasizes the triceps muscles.

Technical Points:
1. Begin exercise with arms fully extended in lockout position.

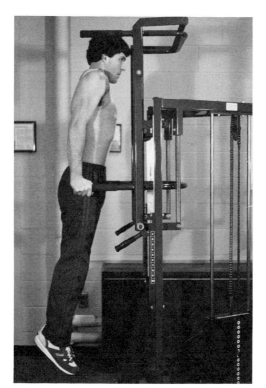

Figure 8–26.   Bar Dip

2. Slowly lower body until upper arms are parallel to floor.
3. Slowly press body upward until arms are fully extended and repeat.

Note: This exercise should be performed with a straight body and a neutral head position. Resistance can be increased by attaching the weightbelt. Persons unable to press their bodyweight should lower slowly and walk back up to the starting position.

BICEPS

The biceps muscles flex the elbows and supinate the hands. The following three exercises are effective for strenghtening the biceps.

Biceps Curl

As presented in Figure 8-27, the biceps curl is a rotary exercise that largely isolates the biceps muscles.

Technical Points:
1. Sit on seat and place elbows on pad in line with machine axes of rotation.
2. Reposition seat or use additional pads as necessary.
3. Hold handles with loose, underhand grip.
4. Slowly lift handles until arms are fully flexed and hold momentarily.
5. Slowly lower handles until arms are extended and repeat.

Note: It is important to keep the elbows on the pad at all times during the exercise. Shoulders should be parallel or slightly lower than elbows. An alternative method of performing the biceps curl is to incorporate the infimetric bar, and work one arm against the other while holding the plates in the top position (see figure 8−28).

Barbell Curl

As illustrated in Figure 8−29, the barbell curl is a rotary exercise that emphasizes the biceps muscles.

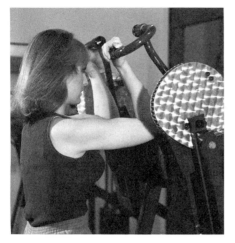

Figure 8–27. Biceps Curl

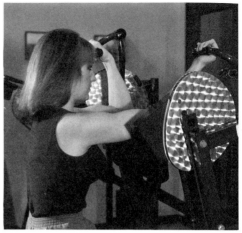

Figure 8–28. Biceps Curl Infimetric Bar

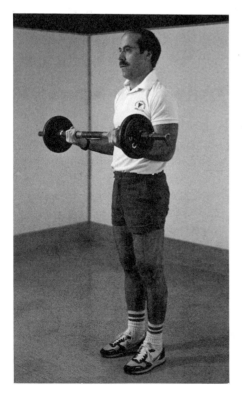

Figure 8–29. Barbell Curl

Technical Points:
1. Hold barbell at full arm extension with a shoulder width, underhand grip.
2. Slowly curl bar to chest level and hold momentarily.
3. Slowly lower bar to starting position and repeat.

Note: It is important to keep the torso erect and the elbows stabilized
against the sides throughout the exercise.

Incline Dumbbell Curl

As shown in Figure 8–30, the incline dumbbell curl is a rotary
exercise that emphasizes the biceps muscles.

Technical Points:
1. Sit on bench with feet on floor.

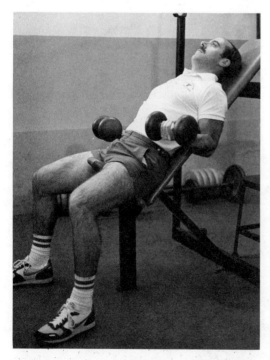

Figure 8–30. Incline Dumbbell Curl

2. Hold dumbbells with underhand grip and arms fully extended.
3. Slowly curl dumbbells to chest level and pause momentarily.
4. Slowly lower dumbbells to full arm extension and repeat.

Note: Hands should be fully supinated in top position for maximum biceps contraction.

NECK FLEXORS

The neck flexor muscles move the chin towards the chest. The neck flexion exercise seems to best isolate this muscle group.

Neck Flexion

As presented in Figure 8–31, the neck flexion is a rotary exercise about the cervical vertebrae.

Technical Points:
1. Sit on seat and place face in center of head pads.
2. Reposition seat or use additional pads as necessary.
3. Place hands loosely on handgrips.
4. Slowly move head forward until neck is fully flexed and pause momentarily.

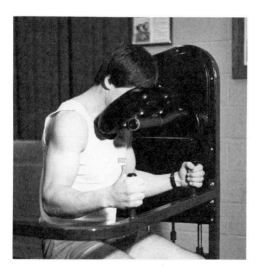

Figure 8–31. Neck Flexion

5. Slowly move head backward until neck is comfortably extended and repeat.

Note: It is important to maintain the torso in an erect position throughout the exercise.

NECK EXTENSORS

The neck extensor muscles move the chin away from the chest. The neck extension exercise seems to best isolate this muscle group.

Neck Extension

As presented in Figure 8–32, the neck extension is a rotary exercise about the cervical vertebrae.

Technical Points:
1. Sit on seat and place head in center of head pads.
2. Reposition seat or use additional pads as necessary.
3. Place hands loosely on handgrips.
4. Slowly move head backward until neck is comfortably extended and hold momentarily.
5. Slowly move head forward until neck is fully flexed and repeat.

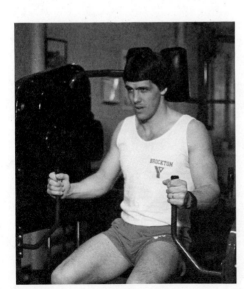

Figure 8–32. Neck Extension

Note: It is important to maintain the torso in an erect position throughout the exercise.

CALVES

The calf muscles extend the ankle joint. The calf raise exercise seems to be effective for strengthening this muscle group. The shin muscles flex the ankle joint. The toe raise exercise addresses this muscle group.

Calf Raise

As illustrated in Figure 8–33, the calf raise is a linear exercise that emphasizes the calf muscles.

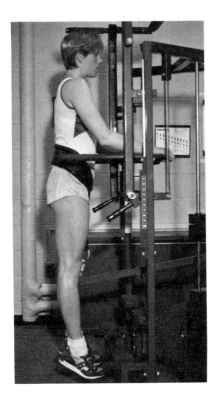

Figure 8–33. Calf Raise

Technical Points:

1. Stand with ball of foot on edge of step.
2. Place weightbelt over hips.
3. Hold handgrips loosely for balance.
4. Slowly lift body until ankles are fully extended and pause momentarily.
5. Slowly lower body until ankles are comfortably flexed and repeat.

Note: Due to the short movement range, it is important to perform this exercise very slowly.

Toe Raise

As shown in Figure 8–34, the toe raise is a linear exercise that emphasizes the shin muscles.

Technical Points:

1. Sit on high table with lower leg in vertical position.
2. Attach weight to toe area with shoestring.
3. Slowly lift toe towards shin until ankle is fully flexed and hold momentarily.
4. Slowly return to starting position and repeat.

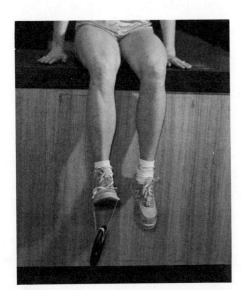

Figure 8–34.   Toe Raise

Note: Due to the short movement range, it is important to perform this exercise very slowly.

FOREARMS

The forearms are involved in all gripping exercises. The forearm extensor muscles extend the wrist, and the forearm flexor muscles flex the wrist. The following is one exercise that stresses both muscle groups.

Wrist Roll

As illustrated in Figure 8–35, the wrist roll is a rotary exercise that emphasizes the forearm flexors during the lifting phase and the forearm extensors during the lowering phase.

Technical Points:
1. Hold roller bar in front of shoulders with overhand grip.
2. Slowly turn roller bar clockwise, alternating left hand and right hand until rope winds weight to top position.
3. Slowly turn roller bar counterclockwise, alternating left hand and right hand until rope unwinds weight to bottom position.

Note: Roller bar should be turned as far as possible with each hand. Rope should not be allowed to slip during the lowering phase.

TRAPEZIUS

The trapezius muscles elevate the shoulder girdle towards the head in a shrugging motion. The shoulder shrug exercise provides an excellent training stimulus to this muscle group.

Shoulder Shrug

As presented in Figure 8–36, the shoulder shrug is a linear exercise that emphasizes the trapezius muscles.

Technical Points:
1. Sit on seat and place forearms palms up between the lifting pads.

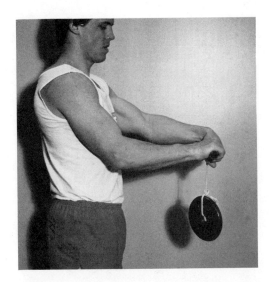

Figure 8—35. Wrist Roll

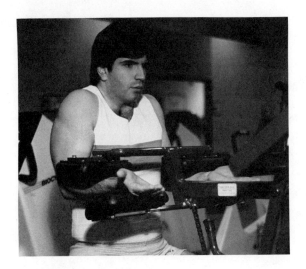

Figure 8—36. Shoulder Shrug

2. Without flexing the arms, slowly elevate the shoulder girdle towards the head and pause momentarily.
3. Slowly lower the shoulders to starting position and repeat.

Note: It is important to maintain the torso in an erect position throughout the exercise.

Chapter Nine

Questions About Strength Training

WHAT RESULTS SHOULD ONE EXPECT?

The development of strength fitness is a complex phenomenon that involves numerous physiological adaptations to imposed training stimuli. When people effectively incorporate the Principles of Stress Adaptation, Rebuilding Time, Near-Maximum Resistance, Controlled Movement Speed, Full-Range Movement, Muscle Balance, and Training Specificity (see Chapter 4), they are almost certain to produce positive physiological adaptations and experience increases in muscular strength. However, it is impossible to predict the rate at which any given individual will gain muscle strength or size. The relationship between strength training and strength improvement is relatively stable over time, but it is rather unpredictable on a day-to-day or even a week-to-week basis.

Table 9–1 presents the rates of strength gain over successive 2½-week training periods for three different training groups (Westcott, 1974). Group A made the greatest increment in strength during the first 2½-week training period. In fact, the rate of strength gain for this group

Table 9−1 Rates of Strength Gain over Successive Two-and-One-Half Week Training Periods for Three Different Training Groups

Training Group	Number	Average Strength Increase during First 2½ Weeks of Training	Average Strength Increase during Second 2½ Weeks of Training	Average Strength Increase during Third 2½ Weeks of Training
A	13	10.6%	6.1%	5.4%
B	20	5.5%	5.7%	4.6%
C	16	6.4%	4.0%	7.2%

was almost twice as high during the first training period as during the second and third training periods. Group B, on the other hand, experienced a relatively even rate of strength development, with the greatest increase occurring during the second 2½-week training period. The response from Group C was also different from that of the other groups. This group achieved a relatively high rate of strength gain during the first training period, a relatively low rate of strength gain during the second training period, and the greatest improvement in strength during the third 2½-week training period. Although Group A is most typical, the rates of strength development for individuals within each of these groups was even more variable, further demonstrating that one's immediate physiological response to strength training is difficult to predict.

Generally speaking, as one continues to train, greater stimulus is required to produce further strength gains. That is, more training stress is necessary to maintain one's muscular progress. A problem arises, however, when greater and greater amounts of stress result in smaller and smaller increments in strength. This state of affairs, often referred to as staleness, is common to athletes in all fitness-related activities. Distance runners and weightlifters are alike in that improvement comes more quickly during the first weeks of practice and less easily as they get closer to their maximum performance potential. For example, a weightlifter who increases his bench press by five pounds a week at the start of his program may improve less than five pounds a year after several years of training, even though the training intensity is considerably greater.

Although it would be nice if everyone's rate of strength gain resembled that displayed in Figure 9−1, a more accurate and realistic represen-

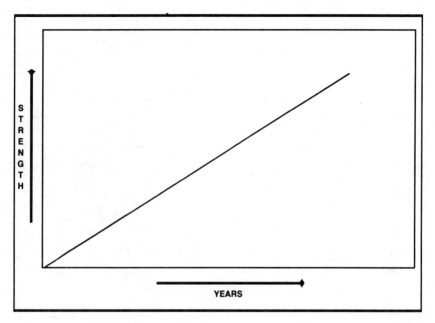

Figure 9−1. Hypothetical relationship between strength development and years of training. In this example, the rate of strength gain remains constant throughout the duration of the training program.

tation of strength development is presented in Figure 9−2. As indicated in the latter figure, the rate of strength gain decreases throughout the duration of one's training career and eventually becomes a rate of strength decrement due to the aging process. The non-training individual begins to lose strength at around age 25, but the person who trains can build strength for many more years and can postpone the loss of strength that inevitably accompanies middle age.

Basically, the principle of diminishing returns applies to the process of strength development. At first, brief workouts result in relatively large strength gains. Later, long workouts produce relatively small increments in strength. For years, weightlifters have rebelled against diminishing rates of strength development by doubling and tripling the length of their training sessions. It is doubtful that this practice significantly increases their rate of strength gain. Unfortunately, extensive workout sessions generally produce the opposite effect. At best, too much stress prevents positive strength adaptations. At worst, it results in chronically fatigued muscles, strength decrement, and tissue injury.

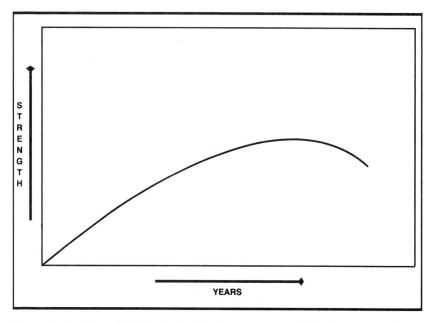

Figure 9−2. Hypothetical relationship between strength development and years of training. In this example, the rate of strength gain decreases throughout the duration of the training program, and eventually becomes a rate of strength loss.

Well-informed exercisers realize that strength gains come more slowly as training continues. They do not fight this natural phenomenon but simply train in harmony with it. They do not expend double the time and energy necessary to achieve optimal progress, but instead increase the exercise intensity. As Darden (1977) has aptly stated, "An advanced trainee does not need more exercise than a beginner; he needs harder exercise and in most cases, less exercise." (page 38).

HOW SHOULD ONE ASSESS PROGRESS?

The key to continued progress is gradual improvement and sensitivity to potential stumbling blocks. The training logbook is an invaluable tool for assessing progress and for correcting small problems before they become major obstacles to strength development. The training logbook should include the date and time of the workout. It should also specify the exercise, the weightload, the repetitions, and any notations such as seat height or technique adaptations. A sample training logbook is presented in Appendix E.

The training logbook provides a systematic means for comparing you to yourself, and that is the only meaningful comparison to make. Comparisons with beginners are usually discouraging because beginners tend to have higher rates of strength gain. Comparisons with advanced trainers are equally discouraging because these individuals have typically attained higher strength levels.

Perhaps the best means of assessing progress is to ask the question, "How does my training today compare with my training four weeks ago?" For such comparison to be meaningful, there must be a degree of consistency in one's training program over a period of time. This is not to suggest that people should never alter a training routine, but that they should stay with a given exercise program long enough for it to be effective. As a rule of thumb, a specific training program should be given a four-week trial period to fairly assess its impact on strength development.

There are basically four variables that should be examined when evaluating a particular strength training program. These are:

1. *Exercises.* Although there are many excellent strength training exercises, it is recommended that one exercise be selected for each of the major muscle groups (see Chapter 8).
2. *Resistance.* Resistance between 65 and 85 percent of maximum is effective for strength development. However, it is suggested that excellent results are obtained when one trains with 70 to 80 percent of maximum resistance.
3. *Repetitions.* While one may train successfully with 5 to 15 repetitions, it is advisable to perform 8 to 12 repetitions per exercise. It is noted that most people can perform 8 repetitions with about 80 percent of maximum resistance and 12 repetitions with about 70 percent of maximum resistance.
4. *Recovery Time.* As the recovery time between exercises decreases, the workout difficulty increases. As a general guideline, one should rest 30 to 90 seconds between exercises, depending on the level of fitness.

One of the best methods for assessing progress is the double progressive training system. The exerciser uses a given resistance and attempts to perform more repetitions each workout. When 12 repetitions are completed, the weightload is increased by 5 percent. The exerciser stays with the new resistance and again works up to 12 repetitions. In this approach, the first variable is repetitions and the second variable is resistance.

It is important to realize that rational decisions regarding a training program can best be made when one utilizes a systematic and progressive approach to strength development. Changing the exercises, resistance, repetitions, and rest periods randomly makes program evaluation difficult. Continued progress is dependent upon the identification and incorporation of those training procedures that seem to be most effective for promoting strength gains. People who train on a day-to-day basis are less likely to discover an optimal training program and more likely to become discouraged with their workouts than people who are consistent and persistent in their approach to strength development.

HOW SHOULD ONE DEAL WITH STRENGTH PLATEAUS?

When progress comes to a halt, one is said to be experiencing a strength plateau. This is sometimes referred to as peaking out, but most strength enthusiasts believe that they can further increase their strength once the cause of the problem is resolved. For the most part, this assumption is correct. The difficulty is in identifying and rectifying the cause of the problem.

It is generally agreed that a strength plateau is an indication that some aspect of the training program should be changed. Such a change usually involves one or more of the following training variables: exercise selection, resistance, repetitions, recovery time, and training frequency. Other considerations may include the type of exercise equipment utilized, the type of diet one is following, and whether to train alone or with a partner.

Although there are numerous factors involved, the basic decision is whether to make one's workout more demanding or less demanding. It has been the author's experience that persons on a strength plateau invariably choose to work harder in an attempt to force further strength development. In most cases, this strategy either maintains the plateau level of strength or results in strength loss. Doing more of the same activity that led to the strength plateau seldom initiates new strength gains. The better alternative is to reduce one's workout demands temporarily to allow the muscle recovery and rebuilding processes to catch up.

Remember that positive muscle adaptations occur during the rest period following the training session. Consequently, the first thing one should do to get off a strength plateau is to schedule more recovery time between workouts. If extended recovery periods do not improve the situation, the exerciser should seriously consider changing the workout routine.

The second consideration is the exercise resistance. For example, the muscles may become so accustomed to 10 repetitions with 75 pounds that this training stimulus no longer promotes positive strength adaptations. If this is the case, switching to 15 repetitions with 65 pounds or 5 repetitions with 85 pounds may make the muscles more responsive.

It is also possible that the exercise intensity must be increased for further strength gains. Let's assume that John has 100 muscle fibers available to perform biceps curls. If he must activate 75 muscle fibers to curl 75 pounds, he alternately switches muscle fibers on and off until 25 of the fibers are fatigued and unable to produce force. At such time, perhaps the 10th repetition, he must discontinue the exercise. However, if John immediately reduces the weightload to 65 pounds he can perform a few more repetitions and fatigue a few more muscle fibers. This training technique, referred to as breakdown training, is a painful but effective way to increase muscle stress and fiber involvement.

If a change in workout intensity does not stimulate further strength gains, it may be necessary to select different training exercises. Many competitive powerlifters have discovered that the best way to get off of a strength plateau in the bench press is to temporarily eliminate this exercise from their training routine. They simply substitute another chest exercise, such as a decline press, an incline press, a Nautilus chest machine, or a dumbbell bench press. After a period of training with the substitute exercise, they return to the bench press and frequently surpass their plateau level of strength after a few workouts.

As indicated in Chapter 8, there are several exercises that can be performed for each of the major muscle groups. Also, any barbell exercise can be effectively executed with dumbbells. The benefit of changing exercises is apparently related to the use of different fibers within a particular muscle group. Different exercises tend to produce different neuromuscular responses, which seem to enhance the overall strength of a muscle. If increased recovery time, different exercise resistance, and greater training intensity have little effect on one's strength plateau, a new exercise may be in order.

Strength plateaus appear to be an inevitable consequence of continued training. Regardless of the training program utilized, there seems to come a time when a change of one type or another is necessary to stimulate further strength development. Strength plateaus should not be cause for discouragement. They are simply reminders that it is time to revise the training routine. It may be an indication for more rest, different resistance, higher intensity training, or new exercises. Whatever changes may be indicated, they should be viewed as positive steps toward one's optimal muscular development.

SHOULD ONE FOLLOW A SPECIAL DIET?

The questions most frequently asked by strength training enthusiasts are undoubtedly those related to diet, particularly the type and amount of protein that should be ingested for optimal muscular development. These are important questions, because proteins are partly responsible for the increased size and strength of trained muscle fibers. In addition to the actin and myosin proteins that form the structural and functional units of skeletal muscle, creatine protein is vital to the process of muscle contraction. Protein is also essential for the formation of bone tissue, blood, and the hormones that influence various physiological processes.

While few people question the importance of protein in the diet, there is considerable disagreement over the amount of protein one should consume on a daily basis, particularly when engaged in heavy strength training activities. The recommended daily protein requirement for adults is one gram of protein for every kilogram (2.2 pounds) of bodyweight. That is, an adult who weighs 90 kilograms (198 pounds) should obtain about 90 grams of protein, which is equivalent to 3.2 ounces of protein. Most Americans consume this much protein in the course of a day simply by following a normal, well-balanced diet. Persons who wish to increase their protein intake can easily do so by eating more protein-rich foods such as milk, yogurt, fish, chicken, peanuts, and soybeans.

The fact is, however, that extra protein generally is not utilized by the body. Neither marathon runners nor weight trainers require additional protein if their daily diet is basically sound. This is true even for persons who are involved in heavy strength training and muscle building activities. It appears that the anabolic (tissue building) processes of the body occur at a relatively constant rate, and are not significantly accelerated by the presence of additional protein. Therefore, optimal muscular development may be obtained without protein supplements, if one adheres to sound nutritional guidelines.

Although there are numerous recommendations concerning training diets and nutritional supplements, there is no research evidence that a good basic diet can be improved upon in terms of enhancing one's muscular development. Such a diet provides the proteins, carbohydrates, fats, vitamins, minerals, and water necessary for optimal health. There are four basic categories of foods that should be included in one's daily meals.

Category 1: Meat-Poultry-Fish-Protein Foods

It is recommended that one obtain at least two servings per day of foods with a high protein content, such as the following:

Beans	Lamb (lean)
Beef (lean)	Nuts
Chicken	Peanuts
Egg whites	Soybeans (Tofu)
Fish	Turkey

Although it is not necessary to eat meat to obtain one's daily protein requirements, it is important to obtain all of the amino acids that are essential for protein synthesis. There are at least 10 essential amino acids that cannot be manufactured in the human body and which must be included in the diet. Meat, eggs, and milk products supply all of these essential amino acids, but no single vegetable, fruit, grain, or nut does so.

Because proteins obtained from animal sources contain all of the amino acids essential for tissue building and repair, they are often referred to as complete or high-quality proteins. Conversely, proteins derived from other food sources do not provide all of the essential amino acids, and are therefore called incomplete or low-quality proteins. It is possible for vegetarians to obtain all of the essential amino acids even though they do not consume meat or dairy products. They must, however, be knowledgeable about the types of proteins contained in their foods and be certain to eat a variety of vegetables, fruits, grains, and nuts to ensure that none of the essential amino acids are excluded from their diet.

Category 2: Dairy Products

In addition to the protein sources discussed in Category 1, it is recommended that one obtain two or more servings of dairy products on a daily basis. The following dairy products are excellent sources of high-quality proteins and calcium, which is a very important nutrient for women.

Cheese (hard)	Skim milk
Cottage cheese (low-fat)	Yogurt (low-fat)
Ice milk	

There has been considerable disagreement regarding the advantages and disadvantages of consuming dairy products when training for muscular strength and definition. The major point of controversy is over the relatively high-fat content of whole milk products. Because skim milk and other low-fat dairy products are readily available in nearly all grocery stores, there does not seem to be any good reason, other than allergic reactions, to avoid this highly nutritious food source. Skim milk furnishes the same amount of protein and calcium as whole milk but has less fat and fewer calories. It is interesting to note that the principal ingredient in most commercially prepared high-protein supplements (powders, pills, and liquids) is non-fat dried milk.

Category 3: Fruits and Vegetables

Fruits and vegetables should make up a large percentage of one's daily food intake. It is recommended that at least four servings in this group be consumed each day. All sorts of fruits and vegetables are included in this category, such as

Apples	Dried fruits
Asparagus	Lettuce
Bananas	Melons
Beets	Onions
Berries	Peaches
Broccoli	Pears
Cabbage	Celery
Carrots	Citrus fruits
Cauliflower	Corn

Peas	Potatoes
Peppers	Squash
Plums	Tomatoes

Although most fruits and vegetable do not have a high protein content, they are generally excellent sources for carbohydrates and for the various vitamins and minerals that are necessary for optimal physical health and athletic performance.

Category 4: Cereals and Grains

Many Americans derive too many calories from some of the foods in this important group. Nonetheless, it is recommended that one obtain at least four servings per day from these food sources. Because it includes breads, pastas, and baked goods, this category is typically the one that people partake of the most. Consider the following food items that are made from cereals and grains:

Biscuits	Pasta
Bran cereals	Pastries
Bread	Rice
Corn cereals	Rice cereals
Crackers	Rolls
Oat cereals	Wheat cereals

Obviously, foods in this category may vary greatly in nutritional and caloric value. Basically, those that are highly refined and comprised largely of white flour, white sugar, and shortening are lower in nutritional value and higher in calories. Examples include cakes, cobblers, cookies, doughnuts, and pies. On the other hand, whole grain products such as dark breads, natural cereals, brown rice, and wheat germ have greater nutritional value and fewer calories. Other grain-based foods such as cereals, crackers, macaroni, and spaghetti fall somewhere in between, depending on the grain source utilized. Many grains and cereals have the additional advantage of providing fiber, which is so important to the efficient functioning of the digestive system.

The person who eats a balanced diet (one that approximates the recommended number of servings from the four basic food groups) should obtain sufficient protein, as well as the necessry vitamins and minerals, to enable maximum gains in muscle size and strength. In other words, protein supplementation is not necessary for promoting muscular gains. On the other hand, although excessive amounts of protein can place a burden on the kidneys, a small increase in one's protein consumption is not physically harmful and may be psychologically helpful to an athlete involved in heavy training. The author can think of few better ways to supplement one's diet, as long as a healthy balance among the four major food groups is maintained. Undoubtedly, a tuna fish sandwich, an apple, and a glass of skimmed milk provides a more nutritious lunch than a bag of potato chips, a candy bar, and a soft drink.

Sample Diet for Bodybuilders

As indicated earlier in this section, proteins are composed of various combinations of amino acids. Because there are 10 essential and 10 non-essential amino acids, some protein foods are of more value than others in tissue building and repair. The best proteins for supplying human growth and maintenance needs are those from animal sources such as eggs, meat, fish, poultry, and milk products. However, because heavy consumption of meat appears to have a relatively high correlation with heart disease and certain types of cancer, it is recommended that several protein sources be utilized in the bodybuilder's diet.

Actually, meat ranks sixth, behind eggs, milk, fish, cheese, and whole grain rice in terms of protein quality. Other excellent sources of high-quality protein include oats, rye, wheat germ, wheat flour, soy flour, peas, beans, potatoes, and spinach. Various nuts, peanuts, and peanut butter are useful protein sources, but they also contain a high percentage of fat.

Of course, bodybuilders need foods from all of the basic food groups to meet their overall nutritional requirements. However, they typically ingest as little fat as possible to reduce subcutaneous fat deposits and enhance muscle definition.

With this in mind, a bodybuilder's breakfast might consist of whole wheat bread, wheat germ with raisins and low-fat milk, low-fat yogurt, and orange juice. For lunch, tuna packed in water, tossed salad with a tablespoon of oil and vinegar, low-fat milk, an apple, and an orange should suffice. The evening meal could include broiled fish with lemon, whole grain rice, sweet potatoes, peas, rye bread without butter, fresh fruit salad, vegetable juice, low-fat milk, and walnut-stuffed dates. Appropriate snack foods could include peanuts, low-fat yogurt, low-fat milk, fresh fruit, or a mixture of rolled oats, raisins, dates, and sunflower seeds.

The sample menu is presented simply as a guideline for obtaining good nutrition while emphasizing high-quality protein consumption and restricting fat intake. It should go without saying that chicken, turkey, lean beef, or veal could be substituted for fish and that a wide variety of fruits, vegetables, whole grains, and low-fat dairy products could be interchanged without disrupting the basic concept of the bodybuilder's diet.

HOW DOES STRENGTH TRAINING AFFECT BODY COMPOSITION?

There has been a widespread misunderstanding regarding the relationship between muscle and fat, particularly with respect to weight training. It is often said that the muscle one develops during the training period will turn to fat once the program is discontinued. This sometimes appears to be the case but actually cannot happen. Muscle is a tissue that tends to get larger when it is used (hypertrophy) and smaller when it is not used (atrophy). Fat is a substance that accumulates in various parts of the body when one's caloric intake exceeds one's energy expenditure. Muscle cannot physically become fat or vice versa.

What frequently happens is this. A person begins a strength training program and experiences muscle hypertrophy. During the training period, caloric intake is increased to meet the new energy and tissue-building requirements of the body. Because the energy demand is equal to the energy supply, fat is not deposited, and the exerciser displays a well-defined muscular physique. Then, when for some reason the strength training program is discontinued, the muscles begin to decrease in size (atrophy). If the caloric intake is not correspondingly reduced to equal the lower energy requirements, fat will begin to accumulate. Consequently, the muscle may be replaced by fat as a result of stopping the exercise program but maintaining the same eating behavior. This phenomenon can be easily avoided by adjusting one's diet to the level of activity or inactivity. When this is done, the individual who stops working out will experience a gradual loss of muscle size and body weight, but will not become fat.

Another misconception concerning weight training is that the training process inevitably makes one bulky. The truth is that many weight-lifters are bulky to begin with, not because they train with weights. For example, a stocky boy or girl may find little success in sports requiring speed, endurance, or agility and may turn to weight training as an alternative activity. The weight training will increase muscle size and strength, but will not, by itself, eliminate a bulky appearance. Only a proper combination of diet and vigorous exercise can produce such a slimming effect. Consequently, one should not assume that a bulky weightlifter looks that way because of the strength training program. More than likely, he or she retains that appearance in spite of the strength training program.

It should be understood that one's basic body build cannot be substantially changed by a weight training program. There is no evidence that strength training can alter skeletal structure or increase the length of one's muscle bellies. Even the degree to which one gains muscle strength and size is genetically determined and regulated through hormone production.

In other words, strength training is limited in application to the muscles being exercised. One can bulk up by lifitng weights and overeating, and one can slim down by lifting weights and undereating, but large changes in body weight are more likely the result of eating patterns than strength training programs.

If one is concerned with both losing fat and building muscle, then strength training is the ideal activity. Although aerobic activity (e.g., running, cycling, swimming) burns many calories, it does not increase muscle mass. These activities have a single reducing effect, because they burn calories while they are being performed (and for a short recovery period following the exercise session).

On the other hand, strength training burns calories and increases muscle density. Because greater muscle mass requires a higher metabolic rate, strength training has a double reducing effect. That is, strength training burns calories during the exercise session *and* during the rest of the day due to the increased metabolic needs of high-density muscles.

This is not to suggest that aerobic activities are less important. Aerobic conditioning is fundamental to physical fitness. However, strength training should be a large part of any fat-loss program. Research (Westcott, 1985d, 1986d) indicates that dieting plus aerobic exercise results in both fat loss and muscle loss, whereas dieting plus strength training results in fat loss and muscle gain. The latter produces beneficial changes in body composition and metabolism that help maintain a lower bodyweight. It is recommended that one follow five guidelines to lose fat in a safe, sensible manner. First, one should eat 3−4 moderate-sized meals per day. Second, one should reduce fat intake to less than 25 percent of the daily caloric consumption. Third, one should reduce daily caloric consumption by 10 percent. Actually, reducing fat intake automatically decreases caloric intake because fats have twice as many calories per gram as proteins and carbohydrates. Fourth, one should perform regular strength training to use more calories and to increase muscle density. Three 20-minute strength training sessions per week are recommended. Fifth, one should perform regular endurance training to burn additional calories and to maintain cardiovascular fitness. Three 20-minute aerobic sessions per week are sufficient, although daily aerobic activity may be preferred.

HOW DOES STRENGTH TRAINING AFFECT FLEXIBILITY?

Flexibility refers to the range of motion in a joint, and has an important relationship to injury prevention and force production. Although an optimum range of joint movement has not been established, a restricted movement range increases the likelihood of injury. Also, joint mobility is an important factor in athletic performance. For example, the greater the distance over which an object is accelerated, the greater the force produced. Consequently, a discus thrower who increases shoulder girdle flexibility will throw farther if all other factors remain the same.

The key to joint flexibility is muscle stretchability, and the key to muscle stretchability is muscle relaxation. Muscle relaxation is the opposite of muscle contraction and represents the absence of tension in the muscle fibers. Muscles possess a property referred to as elasticity. That is, they return to their normal resting length after being stretched. However, if the stretch is sudden, specialized control mechanisms called muscle spindles initiate a stretch reflex that produces a rapid and forceful muscle contraction. This is a protective reaction to prevent the muscle from being damaged by an abrupt or uncontrolled stretching force. For this reason, stretching exercises should never be performed quickly. The preferred way to increase muscle stretchability is to perform slow movements with a short pause in the fully stretched position.

Many people develop a specific stretching program to enhance their joint flexibility. However, properly executed strength training is an effective means for improving flexibility. For example, when the biceps muscle is completely contracted, the triceps muscle is fully stretched. Likewise, when the triceps muscle is completely contracted, the biceps muscle is fully stretched. Consequently, if one trains all of the major muscle groups, one will also stretch all of the major muscle groups. The slow movements that are best for muscle strengthening are also best for muscle stretching.

It should be understood that muscle strength and muscle stretch-ability are different qualities. The former represents a muscle's ability to contract, and the latter represents a muscle's ability to relax. Neither ability has great influence on the other. A high level of strength does not prevent a high level of flexibility, or vice-versa. An exerciser can develop both strength and flexibility through a well-designed and properly executed strength training program.

HOW DOES STRENGTH TRAINING AFFECT SPEED, POWER, AND SPORTS PERFORMANCE?

Speed is an important factor, perhaps the most essential element, for successful performance in many athletic activities. Most sports participants would like to increase their speed of movement (running speed, throwing speed, striking speed, kicking speed, etc.) to enhance their performance level. Unfortunately, as every track coach knows, it is not easy to improve one's movement speed.

Speed is a complex neuromuscular phenomenon. Basically speaking, some people have it and some people do not. Although speed can be improved, no one really knows the best means for doing so. It is generally agreed that speed is most likely to be developed through repeated practice efforts. According to physiologists, repetition of a sports skill increases the probability that the more efficient nerve pathways will become grooved, and that the less efficient nerve pathways will be avoided.

There is actually little relation between speed of movement and strength of movement. That is, one can be strong but not fast, or fast but not strong. Although it is possible and desirable to be both strong and fast, one cannot train for speed and strength simultaneously. In fact, speed training is just the opposite of strength training. It is recalled that the key to strength development is intensity. High-intensity training requires heavy resistance, and heavy resistance prohibits fast movements unless assisting muscle groups are involved.

As an experiment, take a very light barbell and do a curl. Now take a heavy barbell, about the highest resistance you can lift, and again perform a curl. You will not need a watch to convince you that the second lift was considerably slower than the first. Because throwing weights is both a dangerous and a nonproductive procedure, high-intensity strength training must be done slowly.

Speed training, on the other hand, must be performed as quickly as possible to produce the desired results. Because added resistance automatically slows movement time, weight training is not an appropriate means for developing movement speed. For example, let us say that a soccer player wants to increase the speed of his instep kick. He decides to do quick repetitions with 20 pounds in the leg extension exercise to enhance the explosive power of his kicking action. However, kicking a 20-pound resistance is quite different, and much slower, than kicking a soccer ball. Consequently, this type of training is not useful for improving kicking speed. Because the 20-pound resistance is too light to provide any strength benefits, there is little likelihood of producing greater explosive power. In other words, there is little benefit in performing rapid repetitions with light weights. Such exercises use too much resistance for improving speed and too little resistance for increasing strength. They are essentially useless for enhancing athletic performance.

As a second example, consider the shot putter who wants to deliver the shot more quickly. Can fast, lightweight incline presses produce a faster arm action in the shot put? Not unless the weight of the barbell (or dumbbell) is less than the weight of the shot (16 pounds). In fact, even if the resistance were less than 16 pounds, the exercise would probably not improve the speed of the putting action, because the movement patterns are quite different.

How then should one go about developing more speed in the shot put? Certainly not by practicing with a heavier implement, such as a 20-pound shot. In fact, just the opposite approach should be taken. Practicing with a lighter implement (e.g., a 14-pound shot) will permit a faster arm action, which may eventually result in a speedier delivery with the 16-pound shot. The key to improving movement speed is repeated practice using the actual implement (shot, bat, racquet, etc.), or a slightly lighter implement. The use of weight training or heavier than regulation implements is not recommended for developing greater movement speed.

Muscle Power

Speed is quite often equated to power, but speed is only one component of power. Muscle power is actually dependent upon the interaction of three factors: speed, distance, and strength. An increase in the speed of contraction, distance of contraction, or strength of contraction will produce a corresponding increase in power.

In more scientific terms, power is the rate at which work is performed. That is, the amount of work performed during a given period of time is expressed in units of power. The power equation may be written as:

Power = Work/Time

Because work is technically defined as the application of force through a distance, power may also be expressed as the product of force and distance divided by time. This is represented as:

Power = Force × Distance/Time

In accordance with this formula, one may increase power by increasing the movement force, increasing the distance over which the force is applied, or performing the movement in less time.

Although there are several technique-related factors that affect force application (see Appendix B), two physiological factors are basic to the production of muscular force. One is to increase the contractile strength of the muscle fibers, and the other is to increase the number of muscle fibers actively involved in contraction. Both of these physiological responses can be improved through strength training.

Persons with average speed, average range of movement, and average strength can probably attain the greatest increase in power by developing more muscle force. Although speed and flexibility should not be neglected, the potential for greatest improvement typically lies with strength training. As indicated by Westcott's (1985c) study, one can increase muscle strength by about 10 percent after one month of proper weight training.

Strength training for improved power should not take the form of fast repetitions with light resistance. This type of training involves muscle exertion, but does not produce the desired strength adaptations (Westcott, 1985k). Remember that there is a direct relationship between muscle force and power. The most effective means for developing muscle force is high-intensity exercise that incorporates the eight basic strength training guidelines (see Chapter 6).

There are a number of reasons people do strength training, and one of the foremost among these is the desire to improve sports performance. As indicated in a previous section, more strength means more power, and greater power means greater success in most athletic events. Over the past several years, coaches have learned that weight training can increase muscle size and strength without reducing speed and flexibility. Most athletic coaches, therefore, include some form of strength training in their sports programs. Athletes involved in team sports (e.g., football, soccer, basketball, volleyball, baseball, softball, lacrosse, hockey, European handball), dual sports (e.g., tennis, badminton, racquetball, handball, wrestling) and individual sports (e.g., track and field, cross-country, swimming and diving, gymnastics, bicycling, canoeing, golf, archery) can all benefit from well-designed strength training programs.

Persons interested in specific strength training exercises for various sports are referred to Stone and Kroll's book, *Sports Conditioning and Weight Training*. It should be understood, however, that the main purpose of strength training is to increase muscle strength, not to improve athletic skill. Therefore, strength exercises should be selected because they produce desired strength gains, not because they simulate a specific sports movement. Although some outstanding athletes perform resistance exercises that simulate sports skills, they are successful in spite of, rather than because of, this training procedure.

Perhaps the most widespread example of simulated resistance training is swinging a weighted bat. At best, practicing with a weighted bat is a highly inefficient means to increase strength in the contributing muscle groups. At worst, it is a potentially dangerous procedure that could lead to tissue injury. In any case, the slower movement speed experienced when swinging the heavier implement is likely to interfere with the precision timing required when swinging a regulation bat at a 93 mph fastball.

Another common example of simulated resistance training is the use of cables and other devices to imitate various throwing movements (e.g., baseball, football, javelin, discus, shot). There are several problems with this type of training. First, the simulated movement is usually just close enough to the actual skill pattern to confuse the neuromuscular response. Second, the added resistance always results in slower movement speeds. Third, the added resistance is usually insufficient to produce significant gains in strength. Fourth, performing throwing movements with heavier implements or with tethered resistance can place considerable stress on the shoulder, elbow, and wrist joints and may cause injury.

The better approach for improving sports skills is to do strength training for increased muscle force and technique training for better speed and coordination. To be successful, today's athlete must have a high level of strength and a high degree of movement skill. Both abilities are necessary for top athletic performance, and each is best developed through separate and specialized training programs. Every athlete can benefit from a sound program of strength development and a higher level of musculoskeletal fitness.

HOW DO WOMEN RESPOND TO STRENGTH TRAINING?

The average American woman is approximately 4 inches shorter and 30 pounds lighter than the average American man. In addition, she has about 15 pounds more fat weight and about 45 pounds less lean body weight (e.g., muscle, bone, organs). It is therefore not surprising that most females are weaker than their male counterparts. Indeed, strength studies reveal that males typically use twice as much weight in upper body exercises and 50 percent more weight in lower body exercises (Westcott, Benkis, and McPhee, 1985).

Muscle strength is directly related to cross-sectional area. That is, a square centimeter of biceps muscle tissue can produce a specific amount of contractile force, regardless of gender. It therefore follows that a larger biceps muscle is a stronger biceps muscle.

Westcott (1984a) found that previously untrained women increased their arm girth by ¼ inch and their thigh girth by ½ inch after one month of strength training. Because the women experienced no change in bodyweight, the increase in muscle was apparently matched by a decrease in fat.

Due to genetic factors and hormone characteristics, women do not usually increase their muscle size much beyond their first month levels. However, their muscle density may change considerably. In studies utilizing ultrasound measurements of body composition, women have generally increased their muscle mass by about two pounds after two months of strength training (Westcott, 1986d). That is, trained muscles contain less intracellular fat and a higher concentration of muscle fibers. High-density muscles are firm, well-toned muscles that enhance physical appearance and increase metabolism.

Although women rarely develop large muscles, they can certainly develop strong muscles. In fact, due to their lower initial strength, females generally gain strength at a faster rate than males. Westcott (1986j) noted that identical strength training programs produced a 40 percent performance improvement in male subjects and a 70 percent performance improvement in female subjects over the first month of training.

It is important to understand that women can improve their muscle strength and physical appearance through a progressive program of strength training. The only training response difference between men and women is the degree to which muscle strength and hypertrophy are developed. The strength training principles and procedures are identical for males and females, and the same basic exercise program is effective for all persons, regardless of sex or age.

HOW DO PERSONS OVER THIRTY RESPOND TO STRENGTH TRAINING?

Persons over thirty respond to strength training almost the same as persons under thirty. The only difference is the rate of strength gain. During the first two decades of life, the body undergoes muscle growth and development due to normal maturation. Most people retain their strength level during their twenties. After age thirty, the person who does not perform regular strength training experiences a gradual decrease in muscle strength. The rate of strength loss becomes greater during the succeeding decades and is a natural consequence of the aging process. In addition to strength decrement, growing older is accompanied by a decrease in metabolic rate and a reduction in maximum heart rate. Properly performed strength training has a positive influence on the first two degenerative processes. Through progressive resistance exercise, men and women can achieve relatively high strength levels during their thirties, forties, and fifties. Because there is a direct relationship between strong muscles and strong bones, strength training may be particularly useful for older men and women who are subject to decreasing bone density.

Another benefit of strength training is increased muscle density. In addition to producing firmer muscles, this results in a higher metabolic rate due to the increased energy requirements of high-density muscles. As discussed in Chapter 5, every pound of muscle that one develops uses additional calories throughout the day for tissue maintenance and repair.

With the exception of the person who has continued to train during adulthood, one's current strength level can be increased regardless of age. That is, adults who begin a strength training program will experience gains in muscular strength whether they are 35 or 65, and the improved muscle fitness will help them to look better, feel better, and function better.

As a hypothetical example, let's assume that Mr. Jones was an avid weightlifter during his college years, and at that time was capable of bench pressing 300 pounds. After graduation, he discontinued his training program and has done nothing more strenuous than lawn work and recreational sports for the past 20 years. Now, at 40 years of age, he decides to engage in serious strength training once again. He finds that, although he is about 15 pounds heavier than his college weight, he can now bench press only 160 pounds. After four months of training he is able to bench press 220 pounds, and after one year he is up to 270 pounds. Further training maintains but does not increase his strength level. In comparison to his college best, Mr. Jones is only 90 percent (270 lbs./300 lbs.) as strong at 41 years of age as he was at age 20. However, he is 170 percent (270 lbs./160 lbs.) stronger at 41 years of age than he was at 40, and much more fit.

Although a few weightlifters and bodybuilders are still competitive in their forties, the real challenge for most of us is to be the best we can be at the present time. The phenomenal growth of jogging and distance running has in large part been due to the emphasis on self-improvement and a higher level of personal endurance fitness. There is no reason the same motivation should not apply to weight training and strength development. Strength fitness is an important component of physical fitness and should be a desired goal for men and women of all ages.

Critics of strength training often claim that muscular strength is not necessary in today's automated society. That may be true, but then neither is the ability to run 15 miles. The point is that both strength fitness and endurance fitness are worthy goals because they add quality to life. Furthermore, most people who exercise on a regular basis feel better after a session of vigorous muscular activity.

Weight training has been accused of causing damage to the heart and circulatory system due to its strenuous nature. Although strength training may not promote cardiovascular fitness as well as running, cycling, or swimming, it does not appear to be harmful to a healthy individual of any age when performed properly. Proper strength training includes four basic safety factors: (1) using weightloads that can be lifted for about 10 repetitions, (2) continuous breathing throughout the exercise set, (3) controlled muscle movement throughout the exercise set, and (4) loose handgrips. Holding the breath or holding the weight in a given position for more than a moment may occlude blood flow and elevate blood pressure. While these guidelines should be followed by all exercisers, they are a must for persons over 30 years of age and for persons who have coronary risk factors.

Whenever the exerciser reaches a sticking point, the set should be terminated and the weight immediately lowered. Prolonged straining to complete a final repetition or holding the weight in an isometric contraction is not necessary for strength development and is a potentially dangerous procedure for persons with circulatory problems.

With respect to overexertion, weight training may be compared to snow shoveling. Persons who work within their capacity, lifting small loads of snow, should not experience any difficulty in clearing the driveway. On the other hand, persons who struggle to carry as much snow as possible every time they lift the shovel may be headed for trouble. Any all-out effort that produces a prolonged isometric contraction should be avoided whenever possible by persons over age 30.

Because weight training permits a wide range of resistance, it is an excellent strength building activity for persons of all ages. No matter how weak a person may be, the weightload may be adjusted so that 10 repetitions can be completed with appropriate effort. This is not always the case for other strength-related activities, particularly calisthenic exercises (e.g., push-ups, pull-ups, dips) in which only one or two repetitions can be performed.

It is recommended that persons over 30 follow a basic strength training program. They should perform one exercise for each of the major muscle groups and observe the standard training principles and procedures.

Finally, persons over 30 are encouraged to take a total approach to developing and maintaining physical fitness. Some form of endurance activity (e.g., running, swimming, bicycling) should be included to promote cardiovascular conditioning, strength training should be performed to ensure musculoskeletal conditioning, and stretching exercises should be done to maintain joint flexibility. Although the adult who has not been physically active should have a medical check-up before beginning a vigorous exercise program, it has been aptly stated that a medical examination is perhaps more necessary for the adult who chooses to remain sedentary.

WHAT ABOUT WARM-UPS AND COOL-DOWNS?

There has been considerable controversy over the advantages, disadvantages, or neutrality of performing warm-up exercises prior to athletic events and strenuous exercise sessions. Those in favor of using warm-ups generally believe that the resulting increase in body temperature enhances the physical performance that follows. Those not in favor of warming up counter that increased body temperature is one of the factors that limit athletic performance, particularly in endurance-type activities. In either case, it is interesting to note that most warm-up routines have a very insignificant effect on muscle temperature.

With regard to muscle stretchability, most people can temporarily increase their range of movement after performing stretching exercises. Some people prefer to stretch prior to doing the activity, while others feel that stretching is more useful and/or necessary immediately following activity. If range of movement is an important factor in the performance of the activity, then perhaps the appropriate stretching exercises should be done at the start of the activity.

Activities that require precise movement patterns seem to benefit from prior rehearsal in the form of progressively more forceful trials. For example, baseball pitchers, football quarterbacks, and shot putters invariably warm up with a few easy throws, then gradually increase the intensity until they are throwing at full effort. While this procedure seems to help groove the desired response pattern for movements that require fine motor control, its effect on the performance of gross motor movements, such as most weight training exercises, is not known.

Weightlifters usually perform progressively heavier sets in most of their training exercises. While this may be physiologically beneficial in preparing the muscles for heavier weightloads, it also serves as a psychological aid for building the exerciser's confidence prior to the big lifts. Whichever the case may be, the use of warm-ups does not appear to hinder weight training performance and is regarded by most lifters as a helpful procedure.

If the exercise set consists of 10 repetitions, it is probably not necessary to perform warm-up sets with lighter weights. Under normal circumstances, a weightload that can be lifted 10 times should not cause injury or require special preparation. For example, Alan can complete 10 leg extensions in good form with 100 pounds. He is therefore training safely with about 75 percent of his maximum weightload (see Chapter 5). If each repetition requires 7 seconds, Alan will take almost one minute to perform the first 8 repetitions. During this time, the quadriceps muscles experience a very specific warm-up, and are well prepared for the final 2 repetitions. In other words, by the time the quadriceps muscles exert maximum effort, they have had 60 seconds of progressively more difficult repetitions to stimulate the appropriate physiological adjustments.

Nonetheless, it is probably a good practice to perform several minutes of continuous large muscle activity prior to strength training as an added safety precaution. According to Westcott's (1986g) research, 20 minutes of cycling prior to the strength training workout did not significantly reduce muscle performance.

Although more attention is given to the warm-up process, the cool-down period that follows the workout is very important. Because weight training is a high-intensity activity, large amounts of energy must be supplied to the muscles during contraction. Assuming that most exercise sets take about 60 seconds, part of this energy is supplied through anaerobic glycolysis and produces a fatigue by-product known as lactic acid. The longer the lactic acid remains in the muscles, the longer the recovery and rebuilding process. Because lactic acid is removed from the muscles by the blood, what one does immediately following the training period appears to affect the rate of lactic acid removal.

The person who goes directly from the weightroom to the showers and then relaxes the rest of the day does little to expedite the recovery process. The person who immediately follows the workout with a big meal diverts the blood from the muscles to the digestive area and likewise fails to facilitate lactic acid removal. The person who runs a few sprints, does some vigorous rope jumping, or plays a hard game of handball to complete the workout produces more lactic acid and actually prolongs the recovery process. However, the person who performs 10–15 minutes of moderate activity after the workout is likely to experience a faster recovery. The increased circulation that results from walking, jogging, easy swimming, or bicycling seems to hasten the rate of lactic acid removal. Once this fatigue compound has been eliminated from the muscles, the rebuilding process can proceed with less interference.

Another important aspect of the cool-down is to facilitate blood return to the heart, which reduces the risk of cardiovascular problems, blood pressure escalation, and lightheadedness. To be most effective, the cool-down activity should not be merely an extension of the workout, but should involve several minutes of continuous large muscle activity. The intensity of the cool-down activity should be high enough to produce moderate, but not heavy, breathing. Most of all, it should be enjoyable, something to look forward to at the completion of the workout. A relaxed 15-minute swim is not only a pleasant way to end a training session, but can increase joint flexibility and facilitate the removal of lactic acid from the muscles. The cool-down can mean the difference between leaving the locker room feeling exhausted or feeling invigorated.

WHAT IS THE RELATIONSHIP BETWEEN MUSCLE STRENGTH AND MUSCLE SIZE?

Basically, a larger muscle is a stronger muscle, and a stronger muscle is a larger muscle. In fact, muscle strength is directly proportional to muscle cross-sectional size.

The major physiological response to strength training is an increase in muscle fiber size. As shown in Figure 9−3, trained muscle fibers are larger than untrained muscle fibers. However, Figure 9−3 also illustrates that muscle fibers can increase in size without changing the overall muscle circumference. For example, the soft tissue in an untrained arm may be 75 percent muscle and 25 percent fat. After training, the muscle component may increase to 85 percent, and the fat component may decrease to 15 percent, but the external size may remain the same. This is essentially what Westcott (1985d, 1986d) found in his weight-loss studies. The subjects who reduced fat intake and performed regular strength training lost 10 pounds of fat and gained 2 pounds of muscle during the eight-week program. Although muscle mass increased, the greater fat loss resulted in similar circumference measurements.

Westcott (1984a) found that nondieting subjects made small increases in thigh girth (½ inch) and upper arm girth (¼ inch) during a four-week strength training program. Although the gains in muscle size were clearly related to the gains in muscle strength, they did not fully account for the 70 percent improvement in training performance. As indicated by other research (Westcott, 1985c; Hakkinen and Komi, 1983;

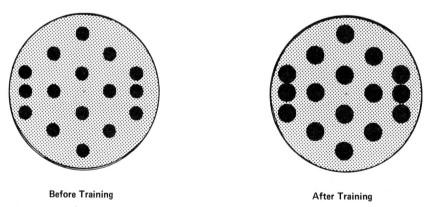

Before Training   **After Training**

Figure 9−3. Schematic Illustration of Increased Muscle Fiber Size Due to Strength Training

Moritani and DeVries, 1979), neurological factors play a major role in strength performance, especially during the early stages of a strength training program. Much of the initial strength improvement is apparently due to better muscle fiber recruitment rather than bigger muscle fiber size.

There are actually a variety of factors that affect muscle strength and muscle size. The type of muscle fibers, the location of tendon insertions, and the length of muscle bellies are inherited characteristics that cannot be altered through training. Consequently, some people have greater genetic potential for developing muscle strength and muscle size.

In the final analysis, it is not always possible to assess muscle strength by external measurements. Because greater muscle strength is accompanied by greater muscle weight, body composition evaluations provide a better means for determining changes in muscle mass. Although not everyone can develop large muscles, everyone can increase muscle density through proper strength training. Perhaps the major objective of a strength training program should be to change weak, low-density muscles into strong, high-density muscles.

WHAT IS THE RELATIONSHIP BETWEEN MUSCLE STRENGTH AND MUSCLE ENDURANCE?

There appears to be a fixed relationship between muscle strength and muscle endurance. As discussed in Chapter 6, if Jim can perform one lift with 100 pounds, he can probably complete 8 repetitions with about 80 pounds and 12 repetitions with about 70 pounds. If John can perform one lift with 200 pounds, he can probably complete 8 repetitions with about 160 pounds and 12 repetitions with about 140 pounds. In other words, most people can perform 8 repetitions with about 80 percent of maximum weightload and 12 repetitions with about 70 percent of maximum weightload. Therefore, as one increases muscle strength, one automatically increases muscle endurance.

During the summer of 1976, the author conducted a simple experiment with his wife. Using the bench press exercise she was tested for her maximum weightload. She was also tested for the number of repetitions she could complete with 45 percent of her maximum weightload. Her training protocol consisted of one set of bench presses, three days per week (see Table 9–2). After six weeks, she was again tested for her maximum weightload and the number of repetitions she could complete with 45 percent of her original maximum weightload. As shown in Table 9–3, her maximum weightload increased from 55 pounds to 70 pounds. This represented a 27 percent increase in muscle strength. Her repetitions with 25 pounds (45 percent of her original maximum weightload) increased from 36 repetitions to 52 repetitions. This represented a 44 percent increase in muscle endurance with a specific weightload.

Although the training program was strictly strength oriented, lasting no longer than 30 seconds per session, the subject experienced a 44 percent improvement in absolute muscle endurance. This result supports a strong relationship between muscle strength and muscle endurance.

From a practical perspective, it would not seem necessary to train for both muscle strength and muscle endurance. It would appear that

Table 9–2   Bench Press Training Program

Week	Monday	Wednesday	Friday
1	45 lb. × 5	45 lb. × 5	50 lb. × 5
2	50 lb. × 5	55 lb. × 3	55 lb. × 3
3	55 lb. × 4	55 lb. × 5	55 lb. × 5
4	60 lb. × 2	60 lb. × 2	60 lb. × 2
5	60 lb. × 2	60 lb. × 3	60 lb. × 4
6	60 lb. × 5	60 lb. × 5	Test Day

Table 9–3   Performance Tests in Bench Press Exercise Before and After 6-Week Training Program

Bench Press Exercise	Before Training	After Training	Percent Increase
Maximum Weightload	55 lbs.	70 lbs.	27%
Maximum Repetitions with 25 lbs.	36 reps.	52 reps.	44%

one automatically increases muscle endurance as one increases muscle strength. For this reason, it is recommended that one follow the strength training guidelines presented in Chapter 6 for improving both muscle strength and muscle endurance.

WHAT IS THE RELATIONSHIP BETWEEN MUSCLE STRENGTH AND CARDIOVASCULAR ENDURANCE?

Muscle strength and cardiovascular endurance represent two extremes on the physical performance continuum. By definition, muscle strength is maximum muscle effort of relatively short duration, and cardiovascular endurance is submaximal muscle effort of relatively long duration. Figure 9–4 identifies a number of activities on the physical performance continuum.

It is possible to have a high level of muscle strength and a low level of

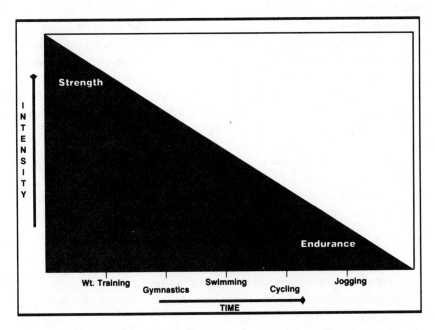

Figure 9–4. Position of various activities along the strength-endurance continuum. Note that strength-related activities are of relatively high intensity and short duration.

cardiovascular endurance, as is typical of many competitive weightlifters. It is also possible to have a high level of cardiovascular endurance and a low level of muscle strength, as is typical of many competitive distance runners. However, it is both possible and advisable to attain relatively high levels of muscle strength and cardiovascular endurance. Ideally, one should have a well-conditioned musculoskeletal system and a well-conditioned cardiovascular system.

The best way to strengthen the musculoskeletal system is through systematic application of the training principles presented in the preceding chapters. The best way to develop cardiovascular fitness is by observing the following training principles established by the American College of Sports Medicine.

Activity. Exercise characterized by sustained, large muscle activity, such as running, swimming, and cycling, is recommended for promoting positive physiological adaptations in the cardiovascular system.

Intensity. The exercise intensity should elevate the participant's heart rate between 60 and 90 percent of maximum. For example, if one's maximum heart rate is 200 beats per minute, the exercise heart rate should be above 120 beats per minute and below 180 beats per minute. Most people receive excellent cardiovascular benefits by training at 75 percent maximum heart rate. In the above example, this would require an exercise heart rate of 150 beats per minute. The maximum heart rate can be estimated by subtracting one's age from 220. That is, a 20-year-old man or woman has an estimated maximum heart rate of 200 beats per minute.

Duration. The target heart rate must be maintained for an appropriate length of time. Depending on the exercise intensity, the exercise duration should be between 15 and 60 minutes. A lower exercise intensity requires a longer exercise duration, and a higher exercise intensity requires a shorter exercise duration.

Frequency. The recommended exercise frequency for developing and maintaining cardiovascular endurance is three to five days per week. The typical cardiovascular fitness program features three nonconsecutive training days per week.

As indicated in Chapter 5, it is possible to meet the criteria for cardiovascular exercise through a "short rest" strength training program in which the participant moves quickly between several exercise stations.

However, this is not the recommended means for achieving cardiovascular fitness. It is suggested that one perform strength training for musculoskeletal development and endurance training for cardiovascular development. Appendix C describes the physiological changes that occur in the heart, blood vessels, blood, and muscles as a result of proper cardiovascular conditioning.

Appendix A

Strength Training Equipment

Further information regarding barbells, dumbbells, Universal Gym, and Nautilus strength training equipment can be obtained by contacting the following addresses:

Nautilus Sports/Medical Industries, Inc.
P.O. Box 1783
DeLand, FL 32720

Universal Gym
Nissen-Universal
P.O. Box 1270
Cedar Rapids, IA 52406

York Barbell Company
P.O. Box 1707
York, PA 17405

Weider Barbell Company
·21100 Erwin Street
Woodland Hills, CA 91367

Appendix B

Principles of Force Production

There are certain basic principles of movement that should be observed when attempting to impart force to an object. The following principles of force production should be understood and applied by athletes involved in dynamic sports events.

Production of Force: To apply maximum force to an object, engage the maximum number of contributing muscle groups.

Direction of Force: To apply maximum force to an object, direct the force through the center of mass of the body and of the object.

Summation of Force: To apply maximum force to an object, begin each successive force at the height of the previous force.

Transfer of Weight: To apply maximum force to an object, move the center of mass in the direction of the force.

Range of Movement: To apply maximum force to an object, accelerate the object over the maximum possible distance.

Speed of Movement: To apply maximum force to an object, accelerate the object in the shortest possible time.

Action-Reaction: To apply maximum force to an object, maintain contact with the ground while the object is being accelerated.

Stretch Reaction: To develop maximum force, precede each muscular contraction with an initial stretch.

Absorption of Force: To absorb an impact, spread the force over the maximum area and the maximum distance possible.

Appendix C

Training Effects of Endurance Exercise upon the Cardiovascular System

Research during the last several years has clearly demonstrated that regular physical exercise of sufficient intensity and duration can produce remarkable adaptations in the cardiovascular system. Beneficial physiological changes take place in the heart, the blood vessels, the blood itself, and the musculoskeletal system. There appears to be an all-or-none law that triggers these internal developments. The three components necessary for cardiovascular improvement are: 1) an exercise intensity sufficient to raise the heart rate to approximately 70 percent of maximum, 2) an exercise duration of at least 15 to 20 minutes and preferably longer, 3) an exercise frequency of at least three nonconsecutive days per week and preferably more often. Although any physical activity that meets these criteria is acceptable, those which are rhythmical and easily controlled (e.g., walking, jogging, bicycling, stationary bicycling, swimming, rope jumping) seem most useful for promoting cardiovascular fitness.

What follows is a partial list of the training effects of an endurance exercise program. In addition to the incredible adaptations exhibited by the cardiovascular system, it is interesting to note that the untrained heart may contract about 40,000 more times per day than the trained heart in order to circulate the same blood volume.

Training Effects

I. Heart becomes a stronger pump.
    A. Stroke volume increases.
    B. Heart rate decreases.
        1. Heart has longer to rest.
        2. Heart has longer to fill with blood.
        3. Heart has longer to receive its own source of oxygen.
    C. Cardiac output increases.

II. Circulatory system becomes more efficient.
    A. Size of blood vessels increases.
    B. Number of blood vessels increases.
    C. Tone of blood vessels increases.
    D. Arterial blood pressure decreases.
    E. Efficiency of myocardial blood distribution increases.
    F. Efficiency of peripheral blood distribution increases.

III. Blood becomes a better transporter.
    A. Number of red blood cells increases.
    B. Mass of red blood cells increases.
    C. Amount of hemoglobin increases.
    D. Amount of plasma increases.
    E. Total blood volume increases (about one quart in average male).
    F. Platelet stickiness decreases.
    G. Levels of triglycerides and cholesterols decrease.
    H. Electron transport capacity increases.
    I. Arterial oxygen content increases.

IV. Other beneficial adaptations.
    A. Glucose intolerance decreases.
    B. Obesity/adiposity decreases.
    C. Thyroid function increases.
    D. Growth hormone production increases.
    E. Vulnerability to dysrhythmias decreases.

  F. Maximal oxygen uptake increases.

  G. Endurance of respiratory muscles increases.

  H. Endurance of locomotor muscles increases.

V. Other possible adaptations.

  A. Improved sleep.

  B. Improved digestion.

  C. Improved elimination.

  D. Improved tolerance to stress.

  E. Improved self-confidence/esteem.

  F. Improved "joie de vivre" including mental and emotional health.

Source: Fox, Samuel M., Naughton, John P., and Gormon, Patrick A. Physical activity and cardiovascular health. *Modern Concepts of Cardiovascular Health* 41(April, 1972): 20.

Appendix D

Strength Training Checklist

The following guidelines are basic to a safe, enjoyable, and effective program of strength development. Review your personal training approach in terms of this checklist.

1. Wear a minimum amount of clothing (i.e., T-shirt, shorts).
2. Wear well-made, supportive athletic shoes.
3. Provide ample space to ensure freedom of movement while performing weightlifting exercises.
4. Engage in a few minutes of warm-up activity (e.g., cycling, rope jumping) before beginning the weight workout.
5. Perform static stretching exercises appropriate for each of the muscle groups that will be stressed during the training session.
6. Lift and lower the weights with a moderate and controlled rhythm.
7. Keep the weights evenly balanced throughout the lifting movements.

8. Inhale and exhale with each repetition. Do not hold your breath when lifting weights.

9. Postpone your scheduled workout if the muscles are still fatigued and recuperating from the previous training session.

10. Attempt to maintain regular training days, but do not train when you are not feeling well (e.g., chest cold).

11. Maintain a weight training notebook for reference and motivational purposes.

12. Whenever possible, train with a partner for safety and encouragement.

13. Try not to compare yourself with others. Remember that each person develops muscular strength at a different rate due to inherent physiological and biomechanical factors.

14. Incorporate jogging, swimming, cycling, or some other endurance type activity into your overall training program. Such activities strengthen the heart and improve the function of the circulatory system to help meet the demands of larger, more active muscles.

15. Performing a few minutes of easy, large muscle activity (e.g., walking, jogging, swimming) after a strenuous weight training workout aids recovery by removing lactic acid from the muscles.

16. For optimal training effects, eat a wide variety of nutritious foods (i.e., meats, fruits, vegetables, dairy products, whole grains and nuts) and obtain ample sleep (seven to nine hours nightly).

Appendix E

Strength Training Logbook

Date _____ Start Time _____ Finish Time _____ Workout Time _____

Exercise: _____   Exercise: _____   Exercise: _____
Weightload: _____   Weightload: _____   Weightload: _____
Repetitions: _____   Repetitions: _____   Repetitions: _____
Notes: _____   Notes: _____   Notes: _____

Exercise: _____   Exercise: _____   Exercise: _____
Weightload: _____   Weightload: _____   Weightload: _____
Repetitions: _____   Repetitions: _____   Repetitions: _____
Notes: _____   Notes: _____   Notes: _____

Exercise: _____   Exercise: _____   Exercise: _____
Weightload: _____   Weightload: _____   Weightload: _____
Repetitions: _____   Repetitions: _____   Repetitions: _____
Notes: _____   Notes: _____   Notes: _____

Exercise: _____   Exercise: _____   Exercise: _____

Weightload: _____   Weightload: _____   Weightload: _____

Repetitions: _____ Repetitions: _____ Repetitions: _____

Notes: _____   Notes: _____   Notes: _____

Rest Period Since Last Workout: _____

Bodyweight: _____

Measurements: _____

Feelings: Strong   Average   Weak
                 Energetic   Average   Tired
                 Enthusiastic   Average   Unenthusiastic

Glossary

Abduction: Sideward movement away from the midline of the body.

Activity Time: Time spent in actual training activity (i.e., performing exercises) as differentiated from time spent in a training facility.

Adduction: Sideward movements toward the midline of the body.

Adenosine Triphosphate (ATP): The chemical compound that, when split, produces the energy for muscular contraction.

Anaerobic Glycolysis: The principal energy source for vigorous activity lasting between 30 seconds and 3 minutes.

Antagonistic Muscle: The muscle that produces the opposite joint action to the prime mover muscle.

Atrophy: Decrease in the cross-sectional size of a muscle.

Berger Program: A system of strength training in which the exerciser performs three sets of 6 repetitions each. All three sets are done with the 6RM weightload.

Bodybuilders: Persons who use strength training as a means for achieving a better muscular appearance, especially with regard to muscle size, shape, definition, and proportion.

Body Composition: The relationship between fat tissue and lean body tissue such as muscle, bone, blood, skin, and organs, Recommended body composition for males is less than 15 percent fat. Recommended body composition for females is less than 20 percent fat.

Bodyweight Exercises: Exercises in which one's bodyweight serves as the resistance. Bodyweight exercises can be augmented by attaching barbell plates to the waist.

Circuit Training: A training program in which one moves immediately from an exercise for one muscle group (e.g., shoulders) to an exercise for a different muscle group (e.g., abdominals), and so on until each major muscle group has been worked.

Concentric Contraction: A contraction in which a muscle exerts force, shortens, and overcomes a resistance.

Controlled Movement Speed: A weightload is raised and lowered in a slow and controlled manner to provide consistent application of force throughout the exercise movement.

DeLorme-Watkins Program: A system of strength training in which the exerciser performs three sets of 10 repetitions each. The first set is done with 50 percent of the 10RM weightload, the second set is executed with 75 percent of the 10RM weightload, and the third set is completed with 100 percent of the 10RM weightload.

Diastolic Blood Pressure: The pressure inside the artery walls during the resting phase of the heart (diastole).

Direct Resistance: The resistive force is applied to the same body segment (e.g., upper arm) to which the movement force is applied.

Eccentric Contraction: A contraction in which a muscle exerts force, lengthens, and is overcome by a resistance.

Endurance: A measure of one's ability to continue exercising with a given, submaximum workload.

Extension: A movement that increases the joint angle between adjacent body parts.

Fasciculi: Groups of muscle fibers bound together by a membrane called perimysium.

Fast-Twitch Muscle Fibers: Muscle fibers that possess a greater capacity for anaerobic energy production.

First-Class Lever: Lever arrangement in which the axis of rotation is between the movement force and the resistance.

Flexion: A movement that decreases the joint angle between adjacent body parts.

Forced Repetition: A spotter can enable the exerciser to complete a lift that would otherwise be unsuccessful by giving a minimum amount of assistance. This procedure for more fully fatiguing the prime mover muscles is referred to as forced repetitions.

Free Weight: Barbells and dumbbells are usually referred to as free weights or loose weights because there are no restrictions on how they are utilized.

Full-Range Movement: Exercising a muscle through a complete range of joint motion, from a position of full extension to a position of full flexion, and vice versa.

Fusiform: Muscles characterized by relatively long fibers that run parallel to the line of pull.

High-Intensity Training: Typically characterized by near-maximum weightloads, as many repetitions per set as possible, and short recovery intervals between successive exercise bouts.

Hypertrophy: Increase in the cross-sectional size of a muscle.

Isokinetic Training: Training on apparatus that automatically varies the resistance in accordance with the applied muscle force. As muscle force increases, the resistance increases proportionately; and as muscle force decreases, the resistance decreases proportionately.

Isometric Contraction: A contraction in which a muscle exerts force but does not change in length.

Lactic Acid: A fatigue-producing by-product of anaerobic glycolysis.

Maximum Heart Rate: The fastest rate that one's heart will contract. Maximum heart rate can be estimated by subtracting one's age from 220. For example, a typical 40-year old man or woman would have a maximum heart rate of 180 beats per minute ($220 - 40 = 180$ beats per minute).

Mini-Gym: One type of isokinetic training equipment that produces accommodating resistance by means of a hydraulic clutch and frictional forces.

Motor Unit: A single motor neuron and all the muscle fibers that receive stimulation from that nerve.

Muscle Balance: Maintaining a natural strength ratio between opposing muscle groups and training for overall muscular development, rather than specializing on particular muscles or exercises.

Muscle Belly: The actual muscle length between the tendon attachments.

Muscle Density: The relationship of muscle tissue and fat tissue within a muscle area. Low-density muscle areas contain large amounts of fat. High-density muscle areas contain small amounts of fat. High-density muscles are stronger, firmer, and have higher energy requirements.

Muscle Fibers: Groups of myofibrils bound together by a membrane called sarcolema, and innervated by a motor neuron.

Muscle Isolation: Designing training exercises so that the movement is accomplished to as large a degree as possible by a single muscle group, such as the Nautilus Multi-Triceps Machine to focus on the triceps muscles.

Muscle Power: Technically, the rate at which work is performed. An increase in the speed of contraction, distance of contraction, or strength of contraction will produce a corresponding increase in muscle power.

Muscle Pump: High-intensity training that saturates the target muscle tissue with blood and temporarily increases the cross-sectional area. This process is often referred to as "pumping-up" the muscles.

Myofibrils: The principal threads running throughout the muscles, myofibrils are formed from adjacent sarcomeres.

Nautilus Equipment: Perhaps the most effective type of strength training equipment, most Nautilus machines provide supportive structure, direct resistance, rotary movement, and automatically variable resistance, which appear to enhance muscle isolation and stress intensification.

Near-Maximum Resistance: Weightloads exceeding 65 percent of maximum are most effective for developing muscle strength and are referred to as near-maximum resistance.

Olympic Lifters: Persons who train with weights in order to lift heavier weightloads in their competitive events, the clean and jerk and the snatch.

One Repetition Maximum (1RM): The heaviest weightload a person can lift once is called the one repetition maximum (1RM) weightload.

Paired Exercises: Following an exercise for a given muscle group with an exercise for the antagonistic muscle group. For example, performing leg curls (hamstrings) upon completing leg extensions (quadriceps).

Penniform: Muscles characterized by relatively short fibers that run diagonally to the line of pull.

Phosphagen: The primary source of energy for vigorous activity of a few seconds' duration.

Powerlifters: Persons who train with weights in order to lift heavier weightloads in their competitive events, the squat, dead lift, and bench press.

Pre-Stretching: A quick stretching (lengthening) of a muscle just prior to contraction that enables the muscle to produce greater force.

Prime Mover Muscle: In any given joint action, the muscle that contracts concentrically to accomplish the movement.

Pyramid Program: A system of strength training in which the exerciser performs successive sets utilizing increasing weightloads and decreasing repetitions. One type of pyramid program consists of 10 repetitions with 55 percent of the 1RM weightload, 5 repetitions with 75 percent of the 1RM weightload, and 1 repetition with 95 percent of the 1RM weightload.

Rebuilding Time: The time required for the muscles to rebuild to a higher level of strength following a training session.

Reciprocal Innervation: The nervous regulatory process that enables an antagonist muscle to relax and lengthen when a prime mover muscle contracts and shortens.

Recovery Time: The rest time allowed for the muscles to partially recover between successive sets of exercise.

Repetitions: The number of times an exercise is performed in succession. For example, the exerciser who takes the barbell from the floor, presses it 10 times, and returns it to the floor has completed one set of 10 repetitions.

Rotary Movement: Movement in a circular pathway, ideally with the resistance axis of rotation in line with the joint axis of rotation.

Sarcomere: The smallest functional unit of muscle contraction, a sarcomere consists of thin actin filaments, thick myosin filaments, and tiny cross-bridges that serve as coupling agents between these two protein structures.

Second-Class Lever: Lever arrangement in which the resistance is between the axis of rotation and the movement force.

Set: The number of separate exercise bouts performed. For example, the exerciser who does 10 bench presses, rests a minute, then does 10 more bench presses has completed two sets of 10 repetitions each.

Six Repetition Maximum (6RM): The heaviest weightload an exerciser can lift 6 times in succession is referred to as the 6 repetition maximum (6RM) weightload.

Slow-Twitch Muscle Fibers: Muscle fibers that have a greater capacity for aerobic energy production.

Spotter: A training partner who gives assistance with an unsuccessful lifting attempt, adds resistance during an exercise, provides encouragement and feedback, and otherwise helps the exerciser train in a safe and effective manner. Spotters should be present in exercises such as the bench press and incline press for safety reasons.

Stabilizer Muscle: A muscle that stabilizes one joint so that the desired movement can be performed in another joint.

Strength: A measure of one's ability to exert muscular force against a resistance.

Strength Plateau: A period of time during which no further strength gains occur. It indicates that some aspect of the training program should be changed to enable further progress.

Strength Quotient: A means of comparing muscle strength among individuals of different sizes. The strength quotient is determined by dividing the maximum weight lifted in a given exercise by the exerciser's bodyweight. For example, a 150 pound person who can bench press a maximum weightload of 300 pounds has a strength quotient of 2.0.

Stress Adaptation: The ability of a muscle to respond positively to progressively greater training demands by gradually increasing contractile strength.

Stress Intensification: Progressively increasing the contractile demands of the muscles by training with more resistance, more repetitions, slower movements, or other means for making the exercise more difficult.

Stretch Reflex: When a muscle is suddenly stretched, specialized control mechanisms called muscle spindles automatically trigger a rapid and forceful muscle contraction known as the stretch reflex or myotatic reflex.

Systolic Blood Pressure: The pressure inside the artery walls during the pumping phase of the heart (systole).

Ten Repetition Maximum (10RM): The heaviest weightload an exerciser can lift 10 times in succession is referred to as the 10RM weightload. Most people can perform 10 repetitions with about 75 percent of their maximum weightload.

Third-Class Lever: Lever arrangement in which the movement force is applied between the axis of rotation and the resistance.

Training Specificity: Training in a specific manner to achieve specific objectives. For example, leg extensions with a 10RM weightload would be more effective for strengthening the quadriceps muscles than a ten-mile run.

Universal Gym: One type of isotonic exercise machine that provides a variety of exercise stations at which smooth running weight stacks are lifted by lever and pulley attachments.

Valsalva Response: Holding the breath during a strenuous lifting movement produces increased pressure in the chest area, which can interfere with venous blood return to the heart and significantly elevate blood pressure.

Variable Resistance Training: Training on an apparatus that automatically changes the resistance throughout the exercise range of movement to accommodate the variations in muscle strength at different joint angles.

Work: The amount of work performed is the product of the force (weightload) multiplied by the distance travelled.

Bibliography

American College of Sports Medicine. 1980. *Guidelines for graded exercise testing and exercise prescription.* Philadelphia: Lea and Febiger.

Astrand, Per-Olof and Rodahl, Kaare. 1977. *Textbook of work physiology, second edition.* New York: McGraw-Hill.

Berger, Richard A. 1962a. Effects of varied weight training programs on strength. *Research Quarterly*, 33:168–181.

Berger, Richard A. 1962b. Optimum repetitions for the development of strength. *Research Quarterly*, 33:334–338.

Berger, Richard A. 1963. Comparative effects of three weight training programs. *Research Quarterly*, 34:396–397.

Berger, Richard A. 1965. Comparison of the effects of various weight training loads on strength. *Research Quarterly*, 36:141–146.

Clark, Nancy. 1985. Calorie adaptations to exercise. *Boston Running News*, 3:14–15.

Clarke, David H. and Manning, James M. 1985. Properties of isokinetic fatigue at various movement speeds in adult males. *Research Quarterly for Exercise and Sport*, 56:221–226.

Clarke, H. Harrison. 1971. *Physical and motor tests in the Medford boys' growth study.* Englewood Cliffs, N. J.: Prentice-Hall.

Clarkson, Priscilla. Muscle physiology and muscle fatigue. Paper presented at Northeast Region YMCA Strength Fitness Seminar, Greenfield, Massachusetts, September 30, 1984.

Darden, Ellington. 1977. *Strength training principles: How to get the most out of your workouts.* Winter Park, Fla.: Anna Publishing Company, Inc.

Darden, Ellington. 1981. *The Nautilus nutrition book.* Chicago: Contemporary Books, Inc.

Darden, Ellington. 1982. *The Nautilus book.* Chicago: Contemporary Books, Inc.

Darden, Ellington. 1985. *The Nautilus book*, revised. Chicago: Contemporary Books, Inc.

DeLorme, Thomas L. and Watkins, Arthur L. 1948. Techniques of progressive resistance exercise. *Archives of Physical Medicine*, 29:263.

Fox, Edward L. 1979. *Sports physiology.* Philadelphia: W. B. Saunders.

Freedson, P., Chang, B., and Katch, F. 1984. Intra-arterial blood pressure during free-weight and hydraulic resistive exercise. *Medicine and Science in Sports and Exercise*, 16:131.

Goldberg, L. E., Schutz, R. and Kloster, F. 1983. Improvement in cardiovascular response to exercise after weight training. *Clinical Research*, 31:9.

Golding, Lawrence A., Meyers, Clayton R., and Sinning, Wayne E. 1982. *The Y's way to physical fitness.* Chicago: YMCA of the USA.

Gordon, H. H. 1967. Anatomical and biomechanical adaptations of muscles to different exercises. *Journal of the American Medical Association*, 201:755–758.

Hakkinen, K. and Komi, P. 1983. Electromyographic changes during strength training and detraining. *Medicine and Science in Sports and Exercise*, 15:455–460.

Hempel, Linda S. and Wells, Christine L. 1985. Cardiorespiratory cost of the Nautilus express circuit. *The Physician and Sportsmedicine*, 13:82–97.

Hettinger, Theodore. 1961. *Physiology of strength.* Springfield, Ill.: Charles C Thomas.

Hunter, G. R. and McCarthy, J. P. 1982. Pressure response associated with high-intensity anaerobic training. *The Physician and Sportsmedicine*, 11:151–162.

Hurley, B. F., Seals, D. R., Ehsani, A. A., Cartier, L. J., Dalsky, G. P., Hagberg, J. M., and Holloszy, J. O. 1984. Effects of high-intensity strength training on cardiovascular function. *Medicine and Science in Sports and Exercise*, 16:483–488.

Ikai, M. and Fukunaga, T. 1970. A study on training effect on strength per unit cross-sectional area of muscle by means of ultrasonic measurement. *European Journal of Applied Physiology*, 28:173–180.

Ikai, M., and Steinhaus, A. H. 1961. Some factors modifying the expression of human strength. *Journal of Applied Physiology*, 16:157–163.

Johnson, LaVon. 1986. The role of muscle in high-level wellness. *The Winning Edge*, 5:1, 5, 12 (March-April).

Jones, Arthur. 1986. Exercise 1986: The present state of the art; now a science. *Club Industry*, 2:36A–64A.

Karpovich, Peter V. and Sinning, Wayne E. 1971. *Physiology of muscular activity.* Philadelphia: W. B. Saunders.

Lamb, David R. 1978. *Physiology of exercise: Responses and adaptations.* New York: Macmillan.

Lamb, Lawrence E. 1985. Understanding calorie use and loss. *The Health Letter*, 27:1–4 (February).

Lesmes, George R., Benham, David W., Costill, David L., and Fink, William J. 1983. Glycogen utilization in fast and slow twitch muscle fibers during maximal isokinetic exercise. *Annals of Sports Medicine*, 1:105–108.

Mathews, Donald K. and Fox, Edward L. 1976. *The physiological basis of physical education and athletics*. Philadelphia: W. B. Saunders.

McDonagh, M. J. and Davies, C. T. 1984, Adaptive response of mammalian skeletal muscles to exercise with high loads. *European Journal of Applied Physiology*, 52:139–155.

MacDougall, J. D. 1985a. Determining factors of strength: Part one. *National Strength and Conditioning Association Journal*, 7:10–23 (February-March).

MacDougall, J. D. 1985b. Determining factors of strength: Part two. *National Strength and Conditioning Association Journal*, 7:10–17 (April-May).

MacDougall, D., Tuxen, D., Sale, D., Sexton, A., Moroz, J., and Sutton, J., 1983. Direct measurement of arterial blood pressure during heavy resistance training. *Medicine and Science in Sports and Exercise*, 15:158.

Messier, Stephen P. and Dill, Mary. 1985. Alterations in strength and maximal oxygen uptake consequent to Nautilus circuit weight training. *Research Quarterly for Exercise and Sport*, 56:345–351.

Micheli, L. 1983. Preadolescents show dramatic strength gains. *The Physician and Sportsmedicine*, 11:25.

Moffroid, Mary T. and Whipple, Robert H. 1970. Specificity of speed and exercise. *Journal of the American Physical Therapy Association*, 50:1692–1699.

Morganroth, J., Maron, B., Henry, W., and Epstein, S. 1975. Comparative left ventricular dimensions in trained athletes. *Annals of International Medicine*, 82: 521–524.

Moritani, T. and DeVries, H. 1979. Neural factors versus hypertrophy in the time course of muscle strength gain. *American Journal of Physical Medicine*, 58:115–130.

Myers, Clayton R. 1975. *The official YMCA physical fitness handbook*. New York: Popular Library.

O'Shea, Patrick. 1966. Effects of selected weight training programs on the development of muscle hypertrophy. *Research Quarterly*, 37:95.

Peterson, James A. 1976. The effect of high-intensity weight training on cardiovascular function. Paper presented at International Congress of Physical Activity Sciences, Quebec City, July 15, 1976.

Peterson, James. 1982. *Total fitness: the Nautilus way*. West Point, N. Y.: Leisure Press.

Pollock, Michael L., Wilmore, Jack H., and Fox, Samuel M. 1978. *Health and fitness through physical activity*. New York: John Wiley and Sons.

Rhoades, Dale and Westcott, Wayne. 1986. Relationships between repetitions and weightloads in bench press and squat. *American Fitness Quarterly*, 6:7–26.

Ricci, G., Lajoie, D., and Petitelerc, R. 1982. Left ventricular size following endurance, sprint, and strength training. *Medicine and Science in Sports and Exercise*, 14:344–347.

Riley, Daniel B. 1982. *Strength training: by the experts*. West Point, N. Y.: Leisure Press.

Schantz, P. 1982. Capillary supply in hypertrophied human skeletal muscle. *Acta Physiologica Scandinavia*, 114:635−637.

Stone, William J., and Kroll, William A. 1978. *Sports conditioning and weight training*. Boston: Allyn and Bacon.

Stone, Michael H., Wilson, G. D., and Blessing, D. 1983. Cardiovascular responses to short term olympic style weight training in young men. *Canadian Journal of Applied Sport Science*, 8:134−139.

Westcott, Wayne L. 1974. Effects of varied frequencies of weight training on the development of strength. Master's thesis, The Pennsylvania State University.

Westcott, Wayne L. 1976. Unpublished research study.

Westcott, Wayne L. 1979. Female response to weight training. *Journal of Physical Education*, 77:31−33.

Westcott, Wayne L. 1984a. Effects of strength training on women studied by YMCA. *Journal of Physical Education and Program*, 81:H8−H9 (December).

Westcott, Wayne L. 1984b. The case for slow weight training technique. *Scholastic Coach*, 54:42−44 (August).

Westcott, Wayne L. 1984c. Modern currents in weight training. *Scholastic Coach*, 54:53 (November).

Westcott, Wayne L. 1985a. The inevitable strength plateau. *Scholastic Coach*, 55:30−31 (September).

Westcott, Wayne L. 1985b. Cardiovascular fitness and strength training. Paper presented at Nautilus National Fitness Seminar, Las Vegas, August 8, 1985.

Westcott, Wayne L. 1985c. Combating disappointment when strength training progress slows. *The Journal of Physical Education and Program*, 81:D14−D15 (June).

Westcott, Wayne L. 1985d. Weight loss and weight gain. *Scholastic Coach*, 55:16−17 (December).

Westcott, Wayne L. 1985e. What happens when the athlete misses a strength workout? *Scholastic Coach*, 54:56−57 (March).

Westcott, Wayne L. 1985f. Determining factors of strength: Part one. *National Strength and Conditioning Association Journal*, 7:10−23 (February-March).

Westcott, Wayne L. 1985g. Determining factors of strength: Part two. *National Strength and Conditioning Association Journal*, 7:10−17 (April-May).

Westcott, Wayne L. 1985h. Instructor training: key to Y fitness leadership. *Journal of Physical Education and Program*, 81:F4−F5 (September).

Westcott, Wayne L. 1985i. Provide steak not sizzle with sophisticated technology. *Journal of Physical Education and Program*, 81:G5−G6 (October).

Westcott, Wayne L. 1985j. Bar dips: the one exercise. *Scholastic Coach*, 54:24 (May-June).

Westcott, Wayne L. 1985k. Power: the critical factor. *Scholastic Coach*, 55:52−53 (August).

Westcott, Wayne L. 1985l. The eight basic principles of muscle strengthening. *Scholastic Coach*, 55:22 (November).

Westcott, Wayne L. 1986a. Muscle development, safety make case for slow strength training. *Journal of Physical Education and Program*, 82:E14−E16 (April).

Westcott, Wayne L. 1986b. Strength training and blood pressure. *American Fitness Quarterly*, 5:38–39.

Westcott, Wayne L. 1986c. Effects of circuit strength training on blood pressure. *American Fitness Quarterly* (in press).

Westcott, Wayne L. 1986d. Losing weight with and without strength training. Paper presented at National YMCA Strength Training Instructor Certification Workshop, San Francisco, Calif., May 1, 1986.

Westcott, Wayne L. 1986e. Comparative effects of two and three strength training sessions per week. Paper presented at National YMCA Strength Instructor Certification Workshop, San Francisco, Calif., May 1, 1986.

Westcott, Wayne L. 1986f. Differences in muscle performance with a given submaximum resistance. *Scholastic Coach*, (in press).

Westcott, Wayne L. 1986g. Integration of strength, endurance, and skill training. *Scholastic Coach*, 55:74 (May-June).

Westcott, Wayne L. 1986h. Comparison of eight repetition training and twelve repetition training with track and field athletes. Paper presented at National YMCA Strength Instructor Certification Workshop, Boston, Mass., April 3, 1986.

Westcott, Wayne L. 1986i. *Building strength at the YMCA*. Champaign, Ill.: Human Kinetics Publishing Company.

Westcott, Wayne L. 1986j. Four key factors in building a strength program. *Scholastic Coach*, 55:104–105.

Westcott, Wayne L. 1986k. Strength training for injury prevention. *Scholastic Coach*, 56:62, 65 (October).

Westcott, Wayne L. 1986l. How many reps per set? *Scholastic Coach*, 56:72–73 (December).

Westcott, Wayne L. 1987. Circuit strength training, an in-season alternative. *Scholastic Coach*, 56:120–121 (January).

Westcott, Wayne L. and Howes, Bernard. 1983. Blood pressure response during weight training exercise. *National Strength and Conditioning Association Journal*, 5:67–71 (February-March).

Westcott, Wayne L. and Warren, Thomas G. 1985. Short rest Nautilus training can improve cardiovascular performance. *Journal of Physical Education and Program*, 81:E18–E19 (July).

Westcott, Wayne L., Benkis, John F. and McPhee, Joseph, 1985. Fitness Evaluation Software. South Shore YMCA, Quincy, Mass.

Wilmore, J. H., Parr, R. B., and Ward, P. 1978. Energy cost of circuit weight training. *Medicine and Science in Sports and Exercise*, 10:75–78.

Withers, R. T. 1970. Effects of varied weight training loads on the strength of university freshmen. *Research Quarterly*, 41:110–114.

Wright, James E. 1978. *Anabolic steroids and sports*. Natick, Mass.: Sports-Science Consultants.

Zohman, Lenore R. 1974. *Exercise your way to fitness and heart health*. Englewood Cliffs, N. J.: CPC International.

Subject Index

Aerobic energy system, 107
Anaerobic energy system, 107
Appearance, 1−2
Athletic performance, 3−4

Injury prevention, 5−6, 101−102

Joint movements
  ankle extension, 25
  ankle flexion, 25
  elbow extension, 21
  elbow flexion, 20
  hip extension, 22
  hip flexion, 22
  knee extension, 21
  knee flexion, 21
  shoulder abduction, 21
  shoulder adduction, 21
  shoulder extension, 21
  shoulder flexion, 21
  shoulder horizontal extension, 22

  shoulder horizontal flexion, 21
  trunk flexion, 22
  wrist extension, 25
  wrist flexion, 25

Lactic acid, 207
Lever arrangements
  first class, 31
  second class, 30
  third class, 28−30

Metabolism, 4−5
Milo of Crotona, 44−45, 47, 50, 52−53,
    55, 57
Momentum, 115
Muscle
  actin filaments, 11−13
  antagonists, 14−15
  ATP, 13
  concentric contraction, 13, 128,
    130−131

Muscle *(continued)*
  density, 202, 209
  eccentric contraction, 14, 128, 130–131, 143
  endurance, 209–211
  energy utilization, 4, 13, 43
  fiber arrangement, 18–19
  fiber types, 18
  force, 3, 15–17, 112
  imbalance, 5–6
  isokinetic contraction, 14
  motor unit, 15–16
  myofibrils, 11
  myosin filaments, 11–13
  physiology, 13
  power, 3, 112, 199–201
  prime movers, 14
  relaxation, 19–20
  sarcomeres, 11
  stabilizers, 15
  strength, 208–211
  stretch, 41–42
  structure, 11

Nutrition
  bodybuilder's diet, 194–195
  cereals, 193
  dairy products, 192
  fish, 191
  fruit, 192–193
  grains, 193
  meat, 191
  poultry, 191
  protein, 190–191, 193–195
  vegetables, 192–193
  vitamins, 191–193

Physical capacity, 2–3
Progress assessment, 186–188

Short rest strength training, 90–93, 121
Strength curve, 141–142
Strength gain, 183–186, 188
Strength plateaus, 38, 188–190

Training effects
  atrophy, 33, 195
  blood pressure, 81–88, 99–100
  body composition, 1, 4, 96–98, 100, 195–197
  cardiovascular performance, 90–93, 100, 211–213
  flexibility, 4, 20, 197–198
  heart rate, 88–90, 100
  hypertrophy, 33–34, 195
  muscle performance, 93–96, 100
  speed, 198–199
  sports performance, 57, 145, 200–202
Training equipment
  barbells, 124, 131–132, 143
  direct resistance, 139–140, 143
  dumbbells, 124, 131–132
  isokinetic, 131
  isotonic, 131
  Nautilus, 14, 105, 124, 126, 137–143
  rotary movement, 138–139, 143
  supportive structure, 137–138, 143
  Universal gym, 132–136, 143
  variable resistance, 140–143
  visible weightstack, 143
Training exercises
  Abdominal Curl, 155–156
  Back Extension, 154
  Barbell Bench Press, 160
  Barbell Curl, 173–175
  Barbell Incline Press, 169–170
  Barbell Squat, 149–150
  Barbell Upright Row, 168–169
  Bar Dip, 160, 172–173
  Biceps Curl, 173
  Calf Raise, 178–179
  Chest Cross, 158
  Dumbbell Rowing, 166
  Duo-Squat, 150–151
  Hip Abductor, 153–154
  Hip Adductor, 152–153
  Incline Dumbbell Curl, 175–176
  Lateral Raise, 167–168
  Leg Curl, 151–152
  Leg Extension, 148–149
  Neck Extension, 177–178
  Neck Flexion, 176–177
  Pull-Down, 165–166
  Pull-Up, 164–165
  Rotary Torso, 156–157
  Rowing Torso, 163–164
  Shoulder Shrug, 180–181
  Super Pullover, 162–163
  10 Degree Chest, 158

Toe Raise, 179–180
Triceps Extension, 170
Triceps Pressdown, 170–172
Wrist Roll, 180
Training factors
  activity integration, 143–146
  age, 36–37, 185, 203–205
  alarm, 41
  Berger program, 66–70
  biomechanics, 27–31
  breakdown training, 110–111, 189
  breathing, 126–129
  continuity, 120–122
  cool-down, 207
  DeLorme-Watkins program, 65–66,
    70
  double progressive program,
    187–188
  duration, 107–109, 122
  exercise selection, 101–105, 122, 187
  experience, 37–39
  forced repetitions, 130
  frequency, 62–64, 98, 105–107, 122
  intensity, 109–111, 122
  negative work, 130
  partners, 129–131
  progression, 118–120, 122
  pyramid program, 68–70

range of movement, 116–118, 122
repetitions, 73–76, 98–99, 187
safety, 123–129
sets, 65–72, 98
sex, 34–36, 202–203
size, 31–34, 208–209
space, 124–125
speed, 76–79, 99, 111–115, 122
technique, 39, 125–126
time of day, 79–81, 99
warm-up, 205–207
Training principles
  controlled movement speed, 39,
    51–52
  full-range movement, 52–54
  muscle balance, 54–56
  muscle isolation, 6, 39
  near-maximum resistance, 50–51
  personal motivation, 6
  rebuilding time, 46–49
  stress adaptation, 44–46
  stress intensification, 6, 39
  training specificity, 40, 56–58

Valsalva response, 128

Weight loss, 4, 96–98, 196–197, 208

Author Index

American College of Sports Medicine,
    92, 212
Astrand, P., 97

Berger, R., 51, 66–70, 73

Clark, D., 112
Clark, H., 37
Clark, N., 96

Darden, E., 70–71, 73, 90, 97, 186
DeLorme, T., 65–70, 73

Fox, E., 92
Freedson, P., 82

Goldberg, I., 90
Golding, L., 96
Gordon, H., 40

Hakkinen, K., 96, 208
Hempel, L., 89–90, 92
Hunter, G., 82
Hurley, B., 90–92

Ikai, M., 41, 96

Jones, A., 73–75
Johnson, L., 97

Lamb, L., 97
Lesmes, G., 79, 112

McDonagh, M., 92, 94
MacDougall, J., 18, 33, 82
Mathews, D., 92
Messier, S., 90, 92, 121
Micheli, L., 37
Moffroid, M., 76

Morganroth, J., 92
Moritani, T., 96, 209
Myers, C., 96

O'Shea, P., 67, 73

Peterson, J., 71, 90, 92

Ricci, G., 92
Riley, D., 71

Schantz, P., 92
Stone, M., 90

Stone, W., 201

Westcott, W., 33–34, 36–37, 48, 51, 62,
        64, 68–70, 72–74, 76–77, 80,
        82, 86, 88–90, 92–94, 97, 99,
        105, 107–108, 121, 144, 183,
        196, 200, 202, 207–208
Wilmore, J., 97
Withers, R., 73
Wright, J., 82

Zohman, L., 90, 121